The Shin Splint Manual

Relief and Protection

Patrick Hafner

Birchbark Publishing

Publisher's Cataloging in Publication

Hafner, Patrick

The shin splint manual: relief and protection / Patrick Hafner

p.   cm.

ISBN-13: 978-0-9801724-0-9

1. Shin splints -- rehabilitation   2. Leg injury -- healing   I. Title

"The natural healing force within each one of us is the greatest force in getting well."

– Hippocrates

Contents

Disclaimer

Consult with your physician before you begin to participate in any workout or exercise program, including exercises in this book. I'm not a medical professional and do not claim to be. I've used all activities and advice listed within, and the described routine helped protect me from shin splints. I have confidence in the enclosed advice and believe it will help you as it did me.

But as required in books of this type, I must state that using the guidelines included in the following pages is done at your own risk.

Introduction

Shin splints.

Even reading those two simple words can evoke pain. If you're here, you either want to determine if you have a case of shin splints, or you already know you do and want to do something about it. Either way, read on.

Any of the following sound familiar to you?

At first a dull aching, just a little tenderness, nipped at your lower legs, specifically your shin area. Either in the front section of your shins, or the back section, or both. Then that annoyance was replaced by occasional piercing pain, these new sensations much more acute than before. The sharp pain then subsided, although the dull aches remained.

Time passed, you pushed through the soreness and continued your activity, and eventually the nagging, dull pain around your shins was replaced by serious surges of discomfort: sharp stabs started to occur, with more intensity and greater frequency. The previously strong, capable muscles along your shins now feel delicate and vulnerable, at times painful to the touch. It has become, in a word, excruciating. But more or less, you continued on with activities.

Then perhaps something along these lines happened. As your lower legs short-circuited with pain, you were forced to cease activity; but even so, the injury lingered. You started to miss out on things: you were maybe on a team, and after the injury commenced, competition took place as you sat and watched. Or you run races, and as a big race – one you'd planned on running – approached, you weren't able to train, fully or at all. You missed that race, and may miss other events that approach on the calendar.

Perhaps you're a fitness enthusiast, and instead of doing your regular workout, you suddenly had no choice but to become inactive, your shins throbbing and your emotions percolating. The whole situation was, and maybe still is, not only physically grueling but emotionally taxing.

Possibly, you tried to jump back in, but things didn't really work out too well. Not at all, in fact; you actually felt more pain. That time it may have actually felt as if muscle was being brutalized, even forcefully separated from bone (it might in fact have been, literally). It almost felt as if cruel ice picks were jabbing in down there. Agony engulfed your shins.

Ughh! The classic understatement when living with full-blown shin splints. But even shouting *ughh* somehow doesn't do the feeling justice.

Ever been subjected to the scenario above? If so, you've likely been, or still are, a victim of shin splints. And there's no need to tell you, it's no fun. Perhaps you're an athlete who covers plenty of ground, be it by running, lunging, scrambling, or hiking. Or at least you used to be, until recently.

And among athletes who run, hike, and scramble on courts and fields, shin splints are generally debilitating and horrendously prevalent. In fact, it is estimated that up to 80% of the 40 million regular runners in America alone will experience some running related injury, with shin splints accounting for over 10% of these.

Runners as a group are particularly susceptible to shin splints; indeed, it is one of the most common overuse conditions among runners. Some researchers have estimated that as many as one in five of today's distance runners have various degrees of shin splint injuries. At one time or another, most runners have felt that hobbling ache somewhere in their shins. In fact, a majority of studies agree that from 5% to 15% of all injures reported by runners are shin splints. Injuries not reported and simply subjected to continued training probably put that percentage much higher.

A recent study reported that shin splints are the most common cause of leg injuries to athletes of all sports. In addition to running, participating in soccer, tennis, basketball, hiking, or any sport that involves running, jumping, or downhill travel can cause shin splints.

Thankfully, the shin splint condition is often preventable. And for those already afflicted, shin splints can be manageable and treatable. Suspect that you have a case of shin splints, and sick and tired of it? Take heart. With proper knowledge and commitment to a handful of simple steps, shin splints are neither inevitable nor everlasting. What to do, and how to do it, is the subject we'll explore here, in order for you to repel shin splints for good. It's mainly a matter of understanding the details about shin splint injuries, as well as how to proceed with your healing process, then committing to it.

Let's take a look.

What Are Shin Splints?

Just what, exactly, constitutes a case of shin splints? What contributes to the debilitating agony this condition so often causes?

To begin with, the catchall term "shin splints" has never had a precise definition; however, it can be described in a nutshell as *chronic shin pain resulting from overuse*.

That's the brief summary of shin splints. In contrast, a detailed discussion of the term "shin splints" focuses on leg pain that occurs below the knee. Specifically, on either the front and outside part of the lower leg, or on the inside section of the lower leg. Overall, the injury is basically inflammation from duress involving the deep tissues of these areas.

But even that makes shin splints sound simple, which they often are not. A case of shin splints can materialize suddenly in a number of different ways. The following details will help explain the main forms that shin splint misery can take, and what factors contribute to it.

Muscle Duress

A common characteristic of shin splints is inflammation of the muscle of the lower legs, referred to by the medical community as *myositis*. The swelling and resulting pain can be primarily a result of microscopic tears in the tissue. These numerous tiny injuries occur as the muscles of the lower leg are either wrenched away from the lining of the bone, or are simply overworked, as injurious activities are repeated over and over.

In addition to overuse injuries involving microscopic tearing and its becoming gradually less intact, the muscle of the shin can be subject to another kind of duress: pressure. The muscle groups of the shin area are enclosed within compartments of protective connective tissue, referred to as *fascia*. The fascia separates different muscle groups from each other. When shin muscles are subjected to exhaustion and ongoing, repetitive overuse, this can cause the fascia tissue to swell, thereby increasing pressure within that fascia's compartment. The muscle – that the fascia is meant to protect – has nowhere to escape, and as such suffers the forces of the swelling within this compartment. Ironically, when it becomes inflamed, the protective tissue housing the muscle can end up injuring the overworked muscle further.

Both the muscle along with its protective fascia covering can become thus traumatized.

TENDON DURESS

Just as embattled muscle can make up a substantial amount of shin splint pain, tendons attached to those muscles may feel similar effects after suffering enough strain.

Muscles on the front of the shin situate close to the bone. The tendons holding these muscles in place are made of thin connective tissue, rugged but not indestructible. The tendons attach where muscle meets bone along the length of the shin. Twists, tugs, pounding, and excessive use can cause these tendons to accumulate wear and tear, as they fight to support and stabilize the function and integrity of the muscles. This buildup of numerous battle scars can result in *tendonitis*; in other words, inflammation of the tendon and/or tendon sheath.

The tendons' attachments to the tibia bone are the focal point of shin splint trauma and fatigue. (More on the bones of the shin just ahead.)

So in addition to pain materializing in muscles of the shin, the injury can also be inflicted upon the very tendons that connect those muscles.

SHIN BONE DURESS

In addition to shin muscles and their related tendons serving as a target for abuse, the bones of the shin themselves can be subjected to trauma and contribute to a bout of shin splints.

There are two main bones in the lower leg: the tibia and fibula. The larger of the two, the tibia, is found on the inner side of the lower leg, and the fibula is located on the outer side. A number of muscles attach to both the tibia and fibula.

Concerning shin splints, the tissues around the tibia bone are the focus. The tibia, which supports more than 80% of the body's weight, withstands the impact and stress from the twisting, bending, and pounding forces generated from running and from numerous other physical activities.

The tissues attached to the tibia are crucial in assisting with these efforts. When these muscles and tendons are overworked – especially when the duress occurs over a long stretch of time – the injurious effects of stress can accumulate, particularly at the points on the tibia bone where these tissues connect.

In order to keep the foot and ankle stable, muscles exert force on the tibia; this force torques away on the tendon attached to the bone. When excessive torque is applied to the shin area, all three tissue types mentioned earlier – muscle, tendon, and bone – are at risk. If the shin area is subjected to such recurring overtraining and abuse, and that pressure on related tissues continues, the nagging pain and inflammation associated with shin splints often follow.

In addition to the punishment exerted by constant torque, shin splint pain can be the result of the tibia enduring impact, such as the hard foot strikes of running. The covering of the bone, a sheath known as the *perisoteum*, may then suffer inflammation. This particular malady is referred to as *tibial periostitis*.

The victim of this tissue irritation usually feels pain on the front of the shinbone, directly under the skin. The tenderness felt from tibial periostitis usually starts about three inches above the ankle and extends up the shinbone approximately three inches or so. It can manifest itself in the form of either mild or severe swelling, usually depending on how soon the person takes action to rectify the condition after it starts.

***

So, shin splints can actually be a combination of conditions: trauma to either the muscles, the tendons, or the bones...or possibly to all three areas at once. What's more, trauma to the involved tissues can take place at one of two muscle insertion points. Consequently, shin splints can occur in two regions of the lower leg, as follows:

ANTERIOR SHIN SPLINTS

The first location is on the front, outside part of the lower leg, technically termed the "proximal anterior lateral region" of the lower leg. Shin splints in this region are sometimes called *lateral shin splints*; lateral shin splints in turn are often referred to by the interchangeable term *anterior shin splints*. From here on we'll refer to duress in this area as anterior shin splints (see Figure 1).

The *tibialis anterior* is the main muscle in the shin area, and the main victim in the case of anterior shin splints. This muscle is used to raise the toes and to push down with the heel of the foot. If you were to stand with feet flat on the floor and then raise up your toes and stand on your heels, you'd be using the tibialis anterior to do this.

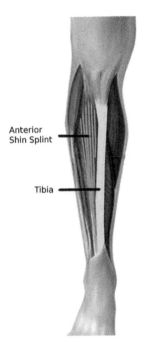

Figure 1: Location of Anterior Shin Splint Trauma

The tibialis anterior muscle is also important for the breaking action of your foot as it hits the ground; if you land on your heels when running, the tibialis anterior absorbs the impact of landing. Landing on the heels is a common method used when runners wear modern, cushioned running shoes; the tibialis anterior in this case would be used extensively. Sometimes too much.

The overuse here is from excessive eccentric loading, such as the absorbing of force described above, on the lower leg's dorsiflexor muscles. This includes the tibialis anterior, as well as other dorsiflexor muscles associated with anterior shin splints. The other dorsiflexors include the *extensor digitorum longus* and *extensor hallucis longus*.

(These details are useful for an overview, but exact muscle names won't be important to remember as you proceed with healing. Thankfully the concepts and steps for recuperation of each muscle in the dorsiflexor muscle group are the same and will be covered just ahead.)

When anterior shin splints make themselves known, the pain will often be first felt when the heel touches the ground during running. The soreness can range from the ankle all the way up to the knee. If excessive strain on the shin region continues even after the injury has begun, the pain could eventually become constant and the shin area tender to the touch.

(**Important Note:** Another overuse condition of the lower leg, called *compartment syndrome*, is sometimes confused with anterior shin splints. The two conditions are different, however. And compartment syndrome is <u>more</u> serious than any type of shin splint. Details regarding compartment syndrome are discussed in the following pages.)

POSTERIOR SHIN SPLINTS

The second location where shin splints can manifest themselves is the "distal medial region" of the leg. Or, specifically, on the inside of the lower leg and the rear of the shin. Shin trauma affecting this area of the lower leg is the most common form of shin splints (see Figure 2).

As if understanding all of this wasn't complicated enough, shin splints occurring in this portion of the leg are referred to by one of three names.

The first term for shin splints affecting the distal medial region is *posterior shin splints*.

The second term, *medial shin splints*, is used in some cases for the exact same condition.

And for shin splints affecting this region, the medical community uses a third term for the condition: *Medial Tibial Stress Syndrome (MTSS)*.

For simplicity's sake, from here on in, we'll refer to the shin splint trauma to the lower leg's distal medial region as MTSS.

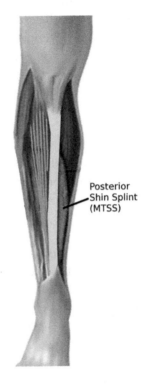

Posterior
Shin Splint
(MTSS)

Figure 2: Location of Posterior Shin Splint Trauma (or MTSS)

When a patient is suffering from MTSS, the tenderness will be present on the inner aspect of the shin. MTSS is typified by pain that starts on the inside of the lower leg above the ankle; the pain becomes worse when standing on the toes or rolling the ankle inward.

The muscle on the back of the lower tibia, the *tibialis posterior*, is especially strained by a case of MTSS. The tibialis posterior wraps around the inner part of the ankle and attaches to the top of the foot's arch. A primary function of the tibialis posterior muscle is to support and hold up the arch of your foot. Each stride you take places stress on the tendons and connective tissues of this muscle. The stress travels up the muscle to its origin on the back/inside of your lower leg.

As a consequence, pain appears on the inner part of the lower leg where the tibialis posterior attaches to the nearby section of the tibia bone. People suffering MTSS may or may not have noticeable swelling over the affected part of the tibia. This type of shin splint will typically be characterized by a dull, nagging, aching pain, but sharp pain can also occur with continued vigorous exertion after the injury has begun.

***

Wow. Muscle, tendon, bone, anterior, and posterior. Got all that? The complete rundown on all shin splint possibilities can be complicated. Luckily, the actions you can take to address the injury are not.

Suffice it to say, the general term *shin splints* can cover a lot of ground, including specifically different forms the injury can take. None of the shin splint types are exactly a joy to live with. Thinking a case of shin splints has already struck? Definitely know that a case of it has? Not quite sure? To determine the presence of shin splints – or not – continue ahead for some clues to self-diagnosis.

Shin Splint Symptoms

Pain from shin splints can vary, even from its early stages. It can range from a dull throbbing to a more intense sensation, on the order of shards of glass being pushed into your tissues. The following types of pain, and areas and conditions in which they occur, may indicate the presence of one or more type of shin splints. Below are some typical shin splint pain characteristics:

- Tenderness or pain along the inside of the shin. It will usually appear about halfway down the shin, but the tenderness may reach all the way up to the knee.

- Tender areas can often be accompanied by one or more small bumps along either side of the shinbone.

– Intense soreness that occurs upon palpitating, kneading, or even gently touching the shin area.

– Shin pain which occurs during exercise or other activity, then reduces with rest. For example, typically the pain is most pronounced at the start of a run, but may recede as the run continues and the tissues get warmed up. However, for runners or walkers on flatter surfaces, this pain can occur at the end of a long outing, usually when the supporting muscles fatigue.

– An increase in pain often when running or walking downhill.

– Shin splint pain is typically progressive. If the injury isn't addressed, and the previous level of exercise or other activity continues, the intensity and duration of the pain usually increases. In cases such as this, running and walking may develop into extremely painful motions. In severe cases, even simple weight bearing may become painful.

– Shin pain that eventually transitions to a constant state, lasting for hours or days after activity. If this happens, you can assume a shin splint condition has set in.

What Causes Shin Splints?

Normal wear and tear over the course of your lifetime *can* contribute to a case of shin splints. The average person takes 5,000 to 12,000 steps daily. In addition to this tremendous number of footfalls, additional twists, stops, starts, and jumps a person may perform over the years can eventually tax the bone, muscle, and connective tissue of the shins. Plus, many of the daily steps a person takes in today's world are on hard, unforgiving surfaces, and each step puts a force on the feet that is about one-and-a-half times that person's body weight. When jogging, your feet and lower legs withstand more than three times this force. Over 10 times your body weight can be incurred while sprinting. During the course of a lifetime, your shins tolerate tremendous workloads as they help and support you while standing, walking, climbing stairs, and running.

Yet, even with all that, the integrity and health of your shin area can remain intact. However, other forces can tip the burden of wear and tear over the edge, forces causing highly repetitive and/or intense strain that can lead to a shin splint injury. Factors such as the following can contribute:

– Excessive pronation (rolling inward of the foot) is a major risk factor for shin splints. When your foot pronates, the muscles must work harder to hold up the arch of your foot, and the tissues of the shin can become unduly stretched and undergo added strain.

– Feet that are either flat or with very high arches.

– A heavy heel strike when running or walking.

– Running on the toes.

– Running with an extremely long stride.

– Running in worn-out and poorly fitting shoes.

– Running on slanted and uneven surfaces. Surfaces that are to either extreme – very soft or very hard – can also encourage shin splints to ensue.

– Running, hiking, or walking steeply downhill, especially when done in a vigorous way and to excess.

– Motions such as sudden stops, starts, and jumps.

– Inadequate strength in the muscles of the lower leg.

– Lack of flexibility in the calf, hamstring, and shin areas.

– A sudden, major increase in the frequency and duration of training. Running is the most common activity in which this occurs, but it can also include long hikes and exercise on machines, as well as rugged manual labor.

– Doing too much total exercise or work without adequate rest, even for the elite athlete. In other words: overtraining and overworking.

– Continuing to exert force on the injured area after warning signs appear…usually with the activities that caused the discomfort in the first place. (Endurance athletes, take note.)

Conditions Sometimes Mistaken for Shin Splints

Conditions other than shin splints can cause shin pain, including *stress fractures* and *compartment syndrome*. The American Medical Association's document titled "The Standard Nomenclature of Athletic Injuries" describes shin splints as pain and discomfort in the leg from repetitive running on hard surfaces or forcible use of foot flexors, with diagnosis being limited to musculocutaneous inflammations, <u>excluding</u> fatigue fracture (in other words a stress fracture) or ischemic disorders (in other words compartment syndrome).

Like shin splints, stress fractures and compartment syndrome are often caused by abuse and overtraining, and at times might feel similar to a shin splint condition. These two conditions are separate injuries from shin splints, though. Let's discuss the important differences.

STRESS FRACTURE

Many people think a stress fracture is simply one type of shin splint, but that's not true. There is quite a difference between shin splints and stress fractures.

A stress fracture is the development of a small crack in those bones that absorb continuous pounding, shock, and other overuse. The presence of such a crack in the tibia bone of the lower leg can be mistaken for shin splints.

Although both conditions are characterized by aching shins, symptoms between a case of shin splints and a stress fracture are usually dissimilar in key ways. With shin splints, pain is most severe at the start of a run, but may disappear during a run as the muscles loosen up. This is different than a stress fracture, where the pain stays fairly constant during just about any weight bearing activity, and the discomfort remains before, during, and after exercise.

Also, pain from a stress fracture is usually specific to a small portion of the bone. This is in contrast to many cases of shin splints, where the tenderness is spread over a greater area.

A couple of theories exist as to why stress fractures manifest themselves. One is based on the bending of related bones due to overload. When the involved muscles contract, they tug and exert stress on the points where they connect to the bone. This stress then causes the bone to bend a bit with each landing. This repeated bend-and-straighten sequence over time generates cracks in the bone.

Another theory suggests that muscle fatigue results in the bone's cracking during a stress fracture. Muscles support both soft tissue and bone, and as the muscles wear down through lengthy exertion or overuse, they can no longer provide the same protection. As the protection the muscles supply gets diminished, the bone bears the greater brunt of impact. Stress fractures can be the result.

If a case of shin splints is not responsive to treatment, a likely next step for a doctor or other medical professional is to examine for stress fracture. Typically the images created by using a bone scan and magnetic resonance imaging (MRI) can determine if the tibia has suffered a stress fracture. Knowing whether a stress fracture is present or not could be crucial: if you continue to exercise with a stress fracture, the injury could eventually lead to a full bone fracture, requiring surgery.

Generally, rest is the key to stress fracture recovery, but complete guidelines for stress fracture recovery are beyond the scope of this book. Think you suffer from a stress fracture? Stress fractures can be hard to self-diagnose, so consult a medical professional and find out for sure.

COMPARTMENT SYNDROME

Compartment syndrome can hurt you and hobble you, and it can also present you with a much more serious situation than a case of shin splints. This debilitating condition often exhibits symptoms similar to shin splints, but occurs for different reasons. Compartment syndrome is realized when pressure within the shin muscles builds to dangerous levels.

Like shin splints, compartment syndrome is most often brought on by excessive exercise or a sudden increase in training intensity. However, a blow, sprain, or contusion endured by the area can also lead to compartment syndrome.

So just what is compartment syndrome? To start with, a covering of tissue forming a closed space, or "compartment," surrounds the muscles on the front of your lower leg near the tibia, specifically the tibialis anterior muscles. Upon being subjected to exertion, these muscles will swell with blood and enlarge. The tissue covering the shin muscles in question will resist this swelling, and as a consequence, pressure builds up within the compartment. This accumulation of pressure can impose on area blood vessels and nerves as well as the muscle, and in turn restrict blood flow to the tibialis anterior muscles. The stymied blood flow along with excessive pressure usually results in severe pain.

Ignoring this pain and pushing on can have tragic consequences. If the pressure of compartment syndrome steadily increases, muscle and nerve damage can occur. The deterioration and trauma leading to permanent damage can occur in less than a day's time, if a present case of compartment syndrome is exacerbated further. If the problem persists and worsens – usually from continued exertion despite the injury – surgery could be ultimately needed.

Compartment syndrome is much more than simple and annoying aches and pains. Take it seriously.

Here are some symptoms of compartment syndrome:

– A dull ache and/or numbed feeling in the large shin muscles on the front and outside of your lower leg. A tingling or numbness could also occur in your feet. If numbness is present in the shins or feet, it's a sign of duress imposed on nerves in the shin area; compartment syndrome often involves pressure on nerves, a case of shin splints will not.

– No increase in pain when stretching. Since it will not increase pressure inside the compartment, stretching will not increase pain in tissues affected by compartment syndrome. Conversely, stretching often will contribute to greater pain in areas suffering from shin splints.

– An increase in pain when exercising. As opposed to shin splints, compartment syndrome pain gets worse during exercise, rather than diminishing as muscles warm up.

– A decrease in pain when resting. Pain from compartment syndrome diminishes greatly or even disappears a short while after exercise ends. The pain from shin splints, in contrast, lingers and sometimes worsens long after the exertion.

Generally, rest is the key to compartment syndrome recovery, but as in the case of stress fractures, treatment and recovery from compartment syndrome are beyond the scope of this book.

But we will say the following: if you're an active person who spends a lot of time on your feet, and you believe you might be suffering from compartment syndrome, cut way back on any activity until you've seen a medical professional. And if you're an athlete who may be afflicted with it: until you're healed, stop training!

A competent medical staff can perform tests to diagnose compartment syndrome by measuring the pressure within the leg compartments before and after exercise. If you have reason to believe you have compartment syndrome, see a medical professional.

Some Medical Treatments for Shin Splints

This book focuses on conservative, low-risk, effective home treatment. But let's first take a look at a few options the medical industry sometimes uses for shin splints. This is an overview, meant to be informative and not exhaustive.

This book does not advocate these treatments, it just describes them. Some folks battling shin splints choose to undergo these methods, others decide against them. To make an informed decision whether any of them are for you or not, consult a physician, ideally one who is familiar with sports medicine.

CORTICOSTEROID INJECTIONS

You may be tempted to seek out a quick fix for your condition, and who wouldn't while suffering from shin splints? That quick fix may appear to you in the form of a corticosteroid injection, which is meant to reduce swelling and pain. The injection often does just that, but its effects are usually temporary. And the temporary relief may come with grave consequences.

The majority of experts agree that corticosteroid injections can come with some nasty side effects. Some of these side effects are as follows:

– Muscle damage in the immediate area.
– Skin pigmentation changes.
– Complete rupture of tendons in the immediate area (as opposed to the much milder strains associated with shin splints).
– Injury to peripheral nerves.
– Atrophy of normal, protective fat layers near the immediate area of the injury.

Repeated injections increase these risks. What's more, the injections are not meant to fix the actual cause of your shin splints, they just temporarily relieve the pain. Use extreme caution before submitting to corticosteroid injections. If you decide to look into corticosteroid injections, you may want to get more than one doctor's opinion.

The position of this book? Don't get corticosteroid injections, ever. They provide temporary relief and never actually fix soft tissue injuries; instead, they often make the injuries worse. In my own run-in with shin splints, I personally chose to stick to conservative home care techniques instead for my bout with the condition. I preferred to address the causes of shin splints rather than simply cover up and temporarily delay its symptoms.

ANTI-INFLAMMATORY AND PAIN MEDICATION

I have strong opinions regarding the popping of pills; my feelings may rub some folks the wrong way, especially in today's somewhat medicated society. In a nutshell, I believe a person should only take pain and anti-inflammatory pills when absolutely necessary, and relying on these meds in an ongoing manner – as if they were a nutrient supplement – is pretty much denying your body's natural abilities to heal, and clutching onto a detrimental security blanket. Maybe an imaginary one at that.

Research backs up my thoughts on this issue. A recent article in the New York Times describes the findings made by exercise scientists at Appalachian State University in Boone, North Carolina. They determined that the healing of injuries to animal tissue when taking NSAIDs (non-steroidal anti-inflammatory drugs), the type of drug compound found in ibuprofen, actually *slowed* the healing of injured muscles, tendons, ligament, and bones. NSAIDs by design inhibit the production of prostaglandins, which are substances that are produced as a reaction to pain. Prostaglandins also help to create collagen, which is the building block of most tissues. So reduced creation of prostaglandins, which NSAID drugs will cause, means less collagen. This will inhibit the healing of injured tissue. Micro-tears and other trauma to muscles and tissues, as in shin splints, fit this category.

If you and your physician decide upon medication to reduce either inflammation or pain, or both, my advice is to take as little of it as you can. As soon as the inflammation is reduced, and sharp pain turns to simple soreness, cease the medication and let your body's natural processes take over. In the case of shin splints, let rest, cold packs, and massage (which we'll cover just ahead) take the place of pills. Of course, that's just my opinion, and it could be debated until the end of time.

Closely related: if you completely numb the pain or soreness of an injury, you may not accommodate it as much as you should with your daily motions and movement. Warning signs like pain and soreness are there for a reason. They may actually help steer you toward optimum injury recovery behavior. Don't dull your senses any more than needed.

In all types of injury recuperation, you need to address what caused the injury in the first place. Pills won't do that for you. For the most reliable, long-lasting recuperation from shin splints, a person should stretch, strengthen, soothe, and accommodate – not medicate.

EXTRACORPOREAL SHOCKWAVE THERAPY

Extracorporeal shockwave therapy uses ultrasound waves to encourage healing, in the hopes that the waves delivered to the affected area promote the creation of new blood vessels and result in better blood flow. It is also theorized that the brain will better "recognize" the injured area after the stimulation, and then send key nutrients to the location to further expedite healing.

Extracorporeal shockwave therapy is a noninvasive procedure, so no cutting will take place. Often an ultrasound image of the injured area is taken, and the medical staff determines the greatest area of pain according to your description.

Then the treatment is delivered using a device that focuses the waves directly on the injured area. No anesthesia is necessary to complete extracorporeal shockwave therapy. Nowadays, the entire procedure can be done in the doctor's office in about 10 minutes. Extracorporeal shockwave therapy has been used now for several years to treat shin splints, and is considered an effective, low-risk procedure.

But please note, in general only the person who has experienced shin splints for several months can opt for this treatment. Medical professionals will first point you to conservative, self-directed therapy...such as that described in this book.

In addition, the conservative therapy shown here will do things extracorporeal shockwave therapy does not do: fix the factors that resulted in your condition. After all, if the underlying causes of shin splint pain remain, the condition can return regardless of your undergoing this procedure or not. Extracorporeal shockwave therapy can be quite costly as well.

What Now?

For anyone who runs, exercises, or even walks and climbs stairs, a case of shin splints can be a serious source of nagging pain. It may be tempting to see a physician or therapist (and if you suspect you have a stress fracture or compartment syndrome, you definitely should). But there's really not a switch that gets flipped if you go to see a medical professional; you aren't likely to leave the first appointment cured.

Conservative home treatment needs to be addressed and considered, whether you seek medical help for shin splints or not. In addition, this kind of approach is most likely what a doctor or therapist will initially advise. The healing process for your injury will need to be established, and then followed. No medical office possesses a magical wand to heal you overnight. A simple, consistent home treatment approach is invaluable for an overuse injury like shin splints, and that's what we'll address in this book.

If you instead do nothing about the injury, and continue to engage in the same activities that caused your case of shin splints, the nagging and sometimes hobbling condition could remain with you for many years. Or it could actually become a chronic malady. Sad to say, but the shin splint condition can in some cases settle in to stay, if abuse of the involved tissues persists.

Don't let it. Before your athletic, fitness, or mobility capabilities completely collapse, take action. Don't allow it to come down to a medical procedure, as listed earlier, as a last resort. Luckily, some of the risk factors listed can be controlled and some behaviors changed to reduce the incidence of shin splints, and to help your body heal. You'll strengthen the structural weaknesses that had helped the injury creep in. Numerous preventive and recuperative options and actions await to help you stave off shin splints; most are rather simple and painless. You just have to learn them, and then do them.

Within this collection of directives, will you discover a magic formula that cures the pain of shin splints instantly? Probably not. There's not one single, simple remedy for shin splints; sometimes a specific motion can really provide relief, but a variety of maneuvers is usually the key. As such, we'll throw the whole kitchen sink at the condition. You'll find several tactics to reinforce the area and make the region's connections strong, resilient, and supple. With these motions and concepts you should enjoy a much higher degree of protection and stability in your shin area.

All action items are non-medical, non-invasive home treatments. They're not risky, and they should not hurt. But following these remedial steps takes perseverance. Each person is unique, as is that person's daily routine, physical condition, bodily structure, and past adventures and misadventures that have resulted in the present level of injury severity. Just a few of the action items may do the trick for you. Or you may need them all. Recuperating from shin splints can be tricky; it's often a fine balancing act, with plenty of inaction as well as action, restraint as well as enthusiasm.

If you're burdened by an injury like shin splints, it's hard to take the fact that your running, playing, walking, hiking, or other exercise regimen has been altered or derailed, or that you can't stay on your feet very long for daily activities. But remember that the sooner you begin, the sooner you will heal, and the more quickly you will get your capable and strong body back.

Make a surge forward and explore the full spectrum of shin splint recuperation and prevention concepts just ahead; resolve to shun the painful condition for good. Nobody knows how long your recovery period will last, but there is definitely one best time to start it: right now. The described actions here are easy, can be done at home, and they work.

Let's get started.

Section 1:
Protect and Defend

The idea of the first phase of this recovery journey is to soothe the shin injury and surrounding tissues, provide some relief from injury-causing factors, and create the best possible atmosphere for your shins to heal. After symptoms of inflammation and acute pain are reduced, it will be safer for you to proceed to the strengthening and stretching activities, which we'll cover soon.

Make a Commitment to Heal and Back Off

Just as important as more active rehab maneuvers is the decision to dedicate yourself to doing whatever it takes to stave off a case of shin splints. To commit. And that commitment includes the willingness to bring certain actions to a halt if that's what it takes to get your shin health back.

Convincing shin soreness to vanish is serious business; you'll have to gird yourself for the challenges ahead, and decide to dedicate a little time and effort to the endeavor. With consistency.

If you have already struggled with the condition for some time, I probably don't need to tell you to commit. If you have just started the process of healing from shin splints, embrace this idea early on, and dedicate yourself to your recovery. The speed with which you heal up is largely dictated by how well you comply with the requirements of rest, not just the active recovery stretching and strengthening motions ahead in the book.

You'll need every advantage you can get. After all, you cannot perform your healing process in a vacuum. You still need to walk, and perhaps climb flights of stairs during the day. You may need to stand on your feet for long periods of time. You might attempt running or other exercise too soon. And each of these and numerous other actions can cause a slight reinjury to your shins; as the reinjuries accumulate, your malady can be prevented from healing in short order. So, you must consistently do many positive things while keeping the negative factors to an absolute minimum. The more the odds can be tipped in your favor, the better.

Most people cannot stay off their feet indefinitely, and this probably includes you. And even if you could, the weakened state of your musculature as a result of this inactivity could end up making matters worse. You must keep moving and stay strong, yet stave off backward progress. The balance required to reduce the condition and heal from it makes for a delicate scenario.

The shin splint condition has no fix-it pill, no miracle cure, no definite recovery time line, and no single cause that can be blamed for its existence. And shin splints have a nasty habit of recurring once normal activities are resumed. It's going to take a serious commitment from you to bring your shins back to a normal, uninjured condition, and then keep them there.

To be sure, a serious mistake is to try to "run through the pain" when suffering from shin splints. The injury itself exists because there is trauma to the bone and/or surrounding tissue; exerting further strain of the same kind in these areas won't improve things. Forcing it more may worsen the injury and make the pain more severe and possibly permanent.

Some victims of shin splints experience lengthy recoveries, while others see the condition can go away almost overnight. Typically, the slow-to-heal victims delay taking action to rectify their injuries. Or just as risky, they jump back into full, rigorous activity too soon.

For the speediest recovery from shin splints, you must stop doing the activity that you suspect caused it in the first place, or at least reduce that activity as much as possible. If only ceasing activity was that easy. If you love to hike or take long walks, turning your back on these activities can be difficult to endure. If you are a dedicated runner or exercise enthusiast, shelving a program can be grueling. You may feel pent up, cooped up, restless, and unfulfilled. To hang up your exercise ritual, even for a short time, may be unthinkable.

If you work on your feet, you face an even more complex scenario. In some ways, your feet and legs are your fortune, and when adjusting a schedule and job duties with a boss and team members you may or may not experience a smooth transition.

But you must reduce the wear and tear on your shins, and that may mean making some tough choices and significant changes to a routine. At least temporarily. If you do not, you could very likely hinder progress toward your recovery.

Fortunately, shin splints sometimes improve greatly just from extended rest. But that usually takes "intervention" from you to help it along. By doing less, often way less. In other words, veer away from the causative activities as best possible, and rest up. Easier said than done in many cases, but crucial for healing. Make an unwavering commitment to help yourself heal, and you'll get that stability back as soon as possible.

Wear Protective Shoes

To minimize further damage or irritation to your shin area, you will need to plant your feet in a supportive, durable, reliable pair of shoes as soon as possible. Once you've got the shoe piece of the puzzle figured out, you'll have made a major stride in activating the healing process.

Along with your shins, good shoes can protect your feet, hips, and back like a dream; bad ones can sabotage them like a nightmare. In fact, dangerous shoes may have landed you and your shins on "injured reserve" list in the first place. The following are some key points regarding ideal shoes and the recovery from shin splints.

Excessive pronation, or *overpronation*, is a common cause of the shin splint injury. Overpronation is generally seen in those who have either flat feet or very bendy, non-rigid feet and ankles. For many aspects of body mechanic safety, flexibility can be a good thing, but in terms of pronation, this excess flexibility may allow foot landings to be unstable. For example, the foot might roll inward at the ankle (see Figure 3), and at the same time the foot's arch could flatten. Therefore, people who have either flat or extremely flexible feet, and thus overpronate as they run and walk, need shoes with a lot of motion control.

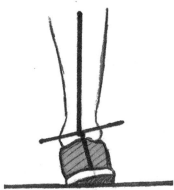

Figure 3: Overpronation of the right foot

A motion control shoe is designed to provide a high level of support, including among other things a very firm midsole and heel counter. The strong midsole is crucial, as a weakening and sagging in a shoe's arch makes the shin's tibialis anterior muscle and its tendon vulnerable to stretches and tears. Good motion control footwear will help to prevent this.

If you overpronate, a motion control shoe is important, but the requirements of an ideal shoe don't end there. Although a sales rep at a reputable footwear store can help you work out the details, here are a few things to look for as you seek new shoes:

- **Stiff Heel Counter.** The back of the shoe where it engulfs your heel should fit firm and snug. Make sure your heel doesn't slide up and down.

- **Flexibility.** Make sure the shoe bends in the front half, where the ball of the foot will be when the shoe is worn. It should not bend in the middle or way back closer to the heel. Your shoe should not bend in any area where your foot does not normally bend. If it does, that shoe's support will be marginal. Conversely, if the shoe barely bends at all, rule it out as an overly stiff shoe that will be detrimental to your feet and lower legs.

- **Proper Fit for Your Feet...Right Now.** Have your feet measured before purchasing your next pair of shoes. Like most parts of our bodies, the feet change with age and the rigors of time. The current shoe size you need may be different than what you wore in the past. The width of your feet should be measured in addition to their length.

- **Arch Support.** Sufficient backbone where the shoe supports your arch is critical. Ensure that the shoe is not flimsy in this area and does not flatten out as you walk.

- **A Little Room to Move.** You'll want a small amount of space in your shoes, both in terms of length and width, so your feet will be comfortable and blood can flow easily. Make sure your new shoes are not too roomy but not too tight either. This is especially important because your feet will swell slightly as the day progresses and the longer you're on your feet. As a matter of fact, for this very reason the best time to try on a pair of shoes is later in the day.

- **A Design Matching High-Arched or Low-Arched Feet.**
  As mentioned above, if you have a low arch, your foot type
  will benefit from a more rigid shoe with motion control
  design. If you have a high arch, your foot type is somewhat
  stiff and requires more cushioning – but not too much.
  Those shoes with extreme cushioning, like the type with
  inflated air pockets lifting the shoe way up, can actually pose
  a risk factor for developing foot, heel, and shin problems;
  there is just no resemblance to actual human anatomy and
  how it carries out natural movements with shoes sporting
  extreme cushioning through the inflated air pocket concept.
  Avoid this design.

- **A Good Fit and Feel Immediately.** A pair of shoes that
  aligns correctly with your feet should feel comfortable upon
  trying them on. Don't assume that the shoes will break in and
  accommodate your feet with time. They probably won't.

Make sure to replace your worn out shoes. Yes, even your
favorite ones. Favorite old shoes, even those with no support left in
them, can be set aside for a while and then somehow find their way
back onto injured, recuperating legs. Acquiring new, solid-performing
shoes is half of the footwear equation. Banish the old faithful but
beat up shoes; they can put your shins back in danger. Throw them
away if they appear to be mostly degraded. If they seem to be in
usable condition but not intact enough for serious exercise, you can
give them away to charity and still feel good about parting ways with
them. And they may in fact work for someone else just fine. It could
be that those shoes are just not right for your feet and circumstances.

For runners, some experts recommend replacing shoes every 500
miles. Other experts say replace them every 300 or 400 miles. For
walkers, add about 100 miles to these figures at most. The owner of
an old and loyal pair can generally tell if support from those shoes is
expiring. If you have a pair of shoes that have served you well, but fit
the description of "waning support," make your peace, bid them
farewell, and get yourself some new ones. Give your shins and all
related muscles, tissues, and joints a new start.

Experiment with Heel Cups

You may want to supplement your new robust, highly protective shoes with a pair of heel cups. A heel cup can be used inside your shoes to control excessive pronation (described in the preceding section), and can be a positive addition to a program of shin recuperation.

A heel cup is simply an insert that is placed inside the back of your shoe to add cushioning and lift your heel a bit. The slight lift a heel cup provides may relieve some of the tension your shin undergoes, and spare it from excessive stretching. (Note: go for a very slight lift – don't choose a heel cup that adds an entire inch to your height or anything close to such a big lift; a half-inch or less is more advisable.) The relief from the heel cup's tiny lift can set up a better environment for shin splint recuperation.

In addition, the cup will supply some mild cushioning. The human foot is equipped with a padding of fat covering the heel. This padding protects your foot against impact and wear. With time, rigor, and age, however, the padding begins to spread out, and some of its shock-absorbing effectiveness is lost. A heel cup will help compensate for this diminished natural protection. It may also supply cushioning which a given pair of shoes does not have. This additional shock absorption will reduce wear and tear to your shins.

Heel cups can be purchased over the counter, and most every pharmacy and department store seems to carry at least one brand. These orthotic inserts are inexpensive, easily acquired and surprisingly helpful for some people. These simple devices can relieve discomfort, promote healing, and in the future ward off a recurrence of shin splints.

Heel cups may help a little or help a lot. Very little risk is involved in experimenting with them. Note: the tightness of your shoes may need to be adjusted after adding a heel cup. You may want to loosen the laces a bit to accommodate the new protective layer in your shoes. Other than that, place the insert in your shoes, and you're ready to go.

Give a pair of heel cups a try and see what you think. They just might lend some immediate relief, reinforce the natural protection your body provides, and help prevent ongoing shin pain.

Adjust Your Training and Exercise Routine

It will be a complete judgment call as to the level of activity you maintain if you become stricken with shin splints. Only one thing is certain: if you believe you were waylaid by overexertion, as runners, hikers, and other athletes with shin splints generally are, then you need to cut back on your activity.

How much to reduce your normal routine? Nobody can tell you for sure, but if your shin area is inflamed and sore to the touch, it's probably not a bad idea to do next to nothing for a while, at least with motions that may have contributed to the injury. Not a popular statement in endurance athlete circles, but…it may be necessary.

I've come across the advice numerous times that the individual suffering shin splints should cut activity just a bit, like by a mere 10% or so. To that I say dream on. Not trying to be snarky here, but a 10% reduction is pretty light duty. If that's all you need to cut back to become healthy again, I'd think you didn't have a really serious situation in the first place. If, on the other hand, you are wincing when walking, cannot run at all nor descend a hill or stairs without pain, and your shin area is tender to the touch, it's in your interest to reduce rigorous activity, either mostly or completely. Think for the long-term, and don't make a case of shin pain into a permanent condition.

In terms of **prevention**, here are some important rules to follow:

Avoid sudden increases in training:

This is a case where the 10% rule is preached again, but I think it applies here more readily. Regardless of the type of training or activity you do, it's advised by many coaches and fitness trainers to never increase your training by increments greater than 10%. This applies to duration, distance, and intensity. A very good rule to follow overall.

That said, consider increasing your training quantity in even smaller amounts. Athletes and exercisers don't always have to go for "longer, better, faster." Consistency and staying power are often much more important than continually stepping it up. Go with training and activity increases of less than 10%, and you'll be sure to not overwhelm your adaptation to exercise quantity. If you often run or walk a three-mile route, just add a 200-yard distance or a city block now and then, if anything. If you're used to jogging for 45:00, don't think you have to add 4:30 (10%) to your session if you decide to step it up. Just add a minute or two at a time. Be sensible and work up at a modest pace. This will lessen your odds of suffering shin splints.

Avoid excessive hill running:

Or, related to the above concept, suddenly adding hills and inclines to your regimen. Very few things pose the risk of acquiring shin splints as do walking, hiking, and especially running on steep hills. In particular, <u>down</u> them. Aggressive inclines and flights of stairs apply here too. Keep this in mind as you look to prevent the injury from cropping up.

Descending hills stresses the muscle of the front of the shin, the tibialis anterior. The tibialis anterior works almost constantly when you run and walk. It is the main muscle that lifts the front of the foot toward the shin. Its other job is to control the lowering of the forefoot after the heel strikes the ground. This requires an eccentric contraction; in other words, the muscle contracts while lengthening.

Without the tibialis anterior's sturdy and stabilizing eccentric contractions, your foot would slam forcefully to the ground with every landing. On hard surfaces like cold asphalt or concrete, the strain of preventing foot slamming is substantial. In the case of runners, this shin muscle effort is often how shin splints begin. Eccentric contractions of any kind are known to cause muscle soreness after exercise, and some shin muscle soreness after running is normal. But when the duress is ongoing, severe, and coupled with inadequate rest, shin splints can follow. Descending hills and inclines will contribute to the "severe" part of that equation.

I love running up and down hills and steep inclines. It almost makes for the perfect endurance and fitness workout: it increases intensity, provides variety over just running on flat ground, and it builds strength, as if your lower body was being worked with weights as you run. Those facts make the shin splint risk of navigating hills and inclines a sad paradox.

The answer: if injured with a case of shin splints, stop exercising on hills for the short term. Once healthy, tackle hills, inclines, and flights of stairs in moderation, work up to a given duration over time, and ideally perform a thorough warm-up before you engage in these workouts and routes. In addition, bolster your defenses with the stretching and strengthening motions we'll cover soon.

Maintain Low Impact Form

In addition to becoming stronger and more flexible, you'll want to minimize one of the primary enemies of your feet, knees, and shins. That enemy is <u>impact</u>. Here are some ways to do that.

Shorten your stride, whether walking, running, or just moving about. Changing the length with which you step can seem awkward at first, but a short time after consciously adjusting your stride you'll most likely stick to it for good. A short stride feels more efficient and actually helps you move forward faster. It will feel better on your feet, heels, and lower legs. And it will decrease your chance of an additional cumulative stress injury like shin splints.

A heavy heel strike results from a long, reaching stride. More impact on your feet and lower legs is the outcome. A lengthy stride can result in more soreness in your knees, hamstrings, quadriceps, and shins. It is inefficient and actually wastes energy. And the added impact will be brutal on your lower legs. This can really add up if you run, as running produces impact several times your body weight. Although the stress will be realized more intensely if you run, the force upon your heels can be about 1.5 times your body weight even when walking. As opposed to a long, lumbering stride, a shorter stride benefits you when walking also, as it helps minimize the force of impact there as well.

Besides using a shorter stride, practice an ideal foot strike. When either walking or running, you may find it tempting to land on the balls of your feet, or even on your tiptoes. But when you land on the balls of your feet or your tiptoes, you actually stress the shins more. The lower leg muscles suffer a tremendous amount of stress when a runner lands only on the balls of the feet or toes, and forgoes normal heel contact. Landing in this way encourages excessive pronation, and the muscles of the foot and leg overwork in an attempt to stabilize the resulting pronated foot. The repeated stress can cause muscle sprain where the muscle attaches to the tibia. The stress realized during any long walks or distance running while landing on your tiptoes will be felt immediately in the foot, knee, and lower leg. And it won't feel pleasant.

Similarly, you should avoid walking or running on the outside edges of your feet. This foot placement will not let the foot roll forward as it was meant to, and like landing on your tiptoes, will probably compound injuries of the foot and lower leg, including shin splints.

You should still land on your heel with each step – ideally toward the *front* of the heel, right around the middle of the foot. Landing on the middle of the foot goes along with a shorter, controlled stride, and results in better shock absorption. You avoid the excessive force from a strike at the very back of the heel, which is all but impossible to avoid if your stride is more like a long, exaggerated lunge.

Even if you feel a little soreness in the lower leg, let the foot roll forward as it does during non-injured walking and running. Landing with the middle of the foot will assist with an ideal rolling forward motion. And remember, as mentioned, good shoes should protect the injured area of your shins to a large extent. So again, make sure you wear good shoes.

And finally, glide with your feet, don't thump. Let your feet skim just above the ground with each step. Don't raise way up and pound the foot down with each step. If you're one of the countless people who walk and run like this (I myself was one), now is the time to adjust the forceful landing you inflict upon your feet.

I know of what I speak here, because I was one of the greatest offenders. For years, I would bound along when running, reaching as far as I could with each leg. My lead foot would fly way above the ground, and then crash down upon landing. My legs and feet would take a terrible pounding, but I persisted with this self-defeating stride. I actually trained for and ran numerous 8K and 10K races this way. In fact, during downhill sections of some courses, I would leap up and out as much as possible with each step, letting myself become airborne for a moment before crushing impact met each footfall. I figured, why not just let gravity take me? And I wondered why my shins were on fire and my hamstring muscles almost nonfunctional with soreness for days afterward. Not to mention, it seemed like the runners whom I had burst past on the downhill portion, the ones with more relaxed, controlled strides, always seemed to pass me up a short time later.

Having trouble picturing what I mean here? If you've ever watched a major league baseball game, and saw the defenders make a key third out, or better yet a double play, you may have seen the players then proudly bound off the field. Way up, way down, loping along with vitality, thundering down with each step of their heroic all-star jog. It looks impressive, and it's actually kind of fun to run that way.

But if your shins are in the process of healing, restrain yourself. Looking good and feeling good can be two different things. Be good to your feet and to your legs. Keep your stride short. Contact with your midfoot. Keep your feet low to the ground, whisking them along and planting them quickly but gently. You'll walk and run with more efficiency, move just as fast if not faster than before, and expose your body to far less damaging impact.

Avoid Dangerous Surfaces

In short, for the health of your lower legs, be careful where you walk and run. Some hazards are obvious. Others can disguise themselves better, and may even look inviting.

Icy areas represent the most evident example of a dangerous surface. With your feet slipping, sliding, gliding, and floating unpredictably in any direction, icy surfaces can inflict extra damage to your already tender shins. And on those flat icy areas with ice and snow chunks frozen in place, walking can be horrific. Don't attempt to navigate ice-covered areas unless you absolutely have to.

Moving across any type of surface that is uneven will be questionable to the safety of your shins. Running habitually on a cambered or sloped surface is a classic cause of shin splints. Luckily, running or walking in such an area will feel uncomfortable, and you probably would sense that it's not good for your shin area. And you'd be right. The leg in the lower position is subject to undue stress, as it carries an excessive proportion of the load in this situation. Choose relatively even surfaces if you can.

But what about a nice sandy beach, or the local park's big, green expanse of grass? Proceed with caution. Both of these surfaces can actually stress the shins to a great degree. Walking or running in soft, sandy areas can be deceptively rough on your feet, knees, back, and shins. Trudging in the sand will often result in the heel plunging below the level of the forefoot at the moment your weight comes to bear over your entire foot. While the heel is in this negative position, the shin area experiences far more pressure than when walking on level ground: the additional force can actually be three or four times greater. That greater load and unstable footing can reverberate through your whole body, and your shin could be affected. A sandy surface may look alluring, but watch out.

Grassy areas pose a mixed scenario: grass has some positive aspects and some negative ones too. The cushion grass provides is undeniable, and it's mostly a good thing. Not much brutal impact will be realized on grass. On the other hand, lawns and fields of grass are inevitably uneven. Bumps, dips, pieces of litter, roots, and rocks can lie hidden anywhere in grass. As can actual holes made by rodents. So despite the padding grass provides, it is not an optimal surface on which to walk or run when recovering from shin splints.

And of course we all know the reality of unyielding concrete, as that's what most sidewalks consist of. Concrete is unforgiving, absorbing almost no shock from your footfalls. Much better choices for walking are dirt, gravel or wood chip paths, providing they are even and in good condition. Asphalt is actually not a bad surface either, specifically in warm weather. Generally, concrete is about five or six times harsher to your shin tissues than asphalt. And asphalt becomes even more shock-absorbing as the sun heats it and makes it soft. In extreme cold, however, it becomes as unforgiving as concrete.

Beware of hills as well. Like grassy surfaces, traveling on hills contains desirable and not so desirable aspects. The vigorous climbs and descents steep hills provide can build strength, endurance, and muscle tone to a great degree, especially in the very leg and rump muscles you need to solidify for future injury protection. Unfortunately, when traveling downhill the shin is getting stressed, and in some cases strained, as it bears the weight of the rest of your body being lowered down the hill.

On the downhill trip, your ankle goes into a position called *plantar flexion*. The plantar flexion position results in a similar foot strike as when walking on the balls of your feet or toes, which is detrimental to the feet and lower leg at any time, but especially when recovering from shin splints. Add to the fact that your body weight is pounding down with extra momentum thanks to gravity on your descent, and the result is a significant load for your injured area to bear. Walking and especially running on hills can be rough on a shin splint sufferer.

Is there any way to limit the strain from traveling up and down hills? I found one strategy helps above all else: keep your stride short. Don't reach way up when going uphill. And don't step big and allow your weight to crash down on your leading foot when going downhill. Landing on your midfoot will help also, as it keeps your foot more level, and diminishes the extreme position of plantar flexion. If you keep your stride short, striking on the midfoot is much easier to accomplish.

Are you expected to maneuver on completely flat and perfectly forgiving surfaces at all times? Of course not. That would be difficult if not impossible to achieve as you move through your day or go for walks in various areas. Hard or slippery surfaces, small hills, and short but steep inclines occur in most areas, and you can travel on them to a limited extent without a problem. The key to remember is the concept of *cumulative stress*. Shin splints result because of stress, strain, wear and tear occurring over and over from certain damaging factors. Don't let the punishment accumulate. Try to avoid risky areas and steep hills if you can, and certainly don't plan to exercise on them when recovering from shin splints.

Ice the Injured Area

Shin splints are an injury, and like most injuries, swelling occurs in the immediate area. This inflammation will not only increase discomfort, it will limit normal motion and impede the healing process. The most immediate and effective method to reduce the inflammation is to apply ice or another cold source to the injury. Ice or a similar cold source will enhance your healing and deaden some of the pain. It will help remove detrimental fluids and allow nutrients to enrich the injured site. This will encourage the repair process and help your shins heal sooner.

Various methods are available to deliver ice applications to the injury, such as commercial ice packs, a plastic bottle filled with water and allowed to freeze, or ice cubes wrapped in a towel. Another good and very convenient method is to simply use a bag of frozen vegetables. Frozen corn kernels and peas are both ideal, as their rounded shape makes for a comfortable texture when you do the icing. The individual pieces in the bag move freely and will mold to the shape of your injured area. And the bags can be used over and over.

The procedure can be as easy as resting your legs on the floor and placing the frozen veggies on top of the shin area or on the sides of it. You can also place the cold source on the floor, lie on your side, and rest your shin area on top of the cold pack. Unless it causes pain, you can work a gentle ice massage into the treatment by moving your leg against the ice pack, slowly and gently.

Do not apply ice or frozen items directly against your skin. This can cause ice burns and damage to your skin. Place a moist towel between your skin and the cold pack to avoid any such danger.

Do not overdo it with icing. Ice treatment of the tender area for 10 minutes at a given time is usually plenty. You can actually damage the tissue if you ice it excessively. Do the icing twice a day in the early stage of shin splints, or if a reinjury of your shin area ever crops up. Once you're well on your way to healing and soreness starts to recede, once a day should be enough.

Icing will be especially valuable if you have just been on your feet for a long time, or right after walking or running. Do it immediately following these activities for best results.

Speaking of walking, running, and reinjury: if you do at some point jump back into activity with a little too much vigor and suffer a reinjury, make sure to apply ice to the area as soon as you can. The benefit of icing an acute injury diminishes after 48 hours or so. Catch the recurrence in time with ice treatment, and the damage will be greatly minimized.

Keep icing in mind for a convenient, low cost, and effective form of therapy. Sit back, relax, and let your aching shin region chill a bit.

Compress the Injured Area

Compression for injury rehab is used to help limit swelling while supporting the muscles and soft tissue of the injured area. Compression is a noninvasive course of action you might want to consider to speed the healing of your injury.

One way to apply compression to your shins is to tape the injured area – athletic taping – before engaging in any exercise to provide stability and discourage additional inflammation. Athletic taping basically includes wrapping tape in a strategic manner around various joints and sections of the body to protect joints, prevent further injury, and introduce compression. In the case of shin splints, the tape would be applied exclusively to deliver compression.

Athletic taping is not included as a how-to in this book, and here's why. Athletic taping could serve as a useful ally during the time you're building up strength and increasing durability in your lower legs. It may allow you to keep moving and working while staving off further injury. However, we feel that to describe the actual technique of a pretty exact procedure like athletic taping through the pages of a book is inadequate for a person looking to learn the proper technique. It's very important to get athletic taping right, as an incorrect or overly tight application of the tape can be hazardous. We recommend that you have someone in the sports medicine field show you the correct technique in person. Hands-on is really the only effective way.

Be aware, to achieve compression's benefits, you do have a great alternative to athletic taping. And that's to consider a commercial compression sleeve for this purpose. A compression sleeve works by gripping your shin area and thus providing gentle compression forces while firmly supporting the lower leg muscles and soft tissue (see Figure 4). Many therapists believe a modern compression sleeve is just as good as taping for compression. A compression sleeve will protect the tissues and stave off swelling while allowing the muscle to move normally when running and walking.

There are many reputable brands of compression sleeves out there, both in athletic supply retail stores and online. If you're looking to get a recommendation on a particular brand, check with qualified staff at an endurance training store, or with a doctor or therapist. Compression sleeves are simple devices and it's hard to go wrong.

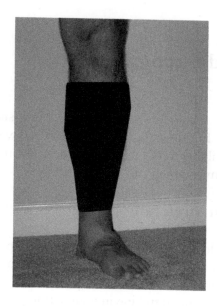

Figure 4: Compression sleeve

So acquire a compression sleeve or learn proper technique for athletic taping from a trainer or therapist. Then let the forces of compression help nurse the tissues of your shin back to health.

Section 2:
Stretch and Strengthen

Tight muscles make the shin work harder as it stabilizes, lowers, and lifts the foot. In this section, we'll explore a few simple methods to encourage flexibility in key areas, ease the tension on your shins, and provide an environment for faster healing.

A Word About Stretching

For starters, do not stretch any region if acute pain exists, or if sharp pain results from stretching motions. If you are in the acute stages of shin splints, where the area is painful to the touch, it may be too early to implement stretching in your action plan. Wait until rest and protection let the area start to recuperate, then try some of the stretches listed with caution in mind. And, just as importantly, if you think you're up for stretching, but a given motion causes sharp pain, cease it immediately. You may not be ready yet.

No absolute verdict has ever been reached on the very best method with which to stretch portions of the human body. If you had the will and unlimited time, and researched the topic until locating 100 articles or books on stretching, I think you would find some glaring discrepancies. It's easy to find 10 or 20 or 30 different takes on the number of repetitions, length of time to hold a stretch, stretching a cold muscle vs. a warmed-up muscle, and how far to stretch an inflexible muscle. Overwhelming agreement amongst the experts on stretching does not seem to exist. And I don't have the final answer on stretching, but I know a couple of things:

Stretching can help you recover from shin splints, and
Stretching can INJURE you further.

Over the years of running races and training, I got into the bad habit of never stretching. My guess is that this lack of stretching helped me acquire overuse injuries in the first place. But once I started stretching on a regular basis, the healing process of these injuries accelerated – greatly. The healing seemed to take place several times faster. And on walks and hikes where the soreness would recur, taking the time to stretch again would usually reduce the pain or make it go away completely. Stretching is a good thing, and most experts on the subject agree that it is not only helpful, but imperative, to stretch in order to resolve a myriad of overuse injuries, including shin splints.

So let me reiterate: I'm all for stretching. A stretching routine helped me come back from shin splints, I.T. Band Syndrome, and a very rough case of plantar fasciitis, and it keeps my feet, heels, and legs safe to this day. Stretching is an integral part of this book and can serve as an invaluable healing mechanism for anyone who suffers from or wants to prevent shin splints.

But if you stretch a muscle with too much force and in too much of a hurry, the muscle can tear. And your injury problem will then become compounded. So keep three words in mind for a successful stretching venture:

Consistent. Patient. Gentle.

When overcoming a case of shin splints, only perform the stretches after warming up. A slow walk that gradually increases to medium speed generally works.

Stretch regularly, at least once a day, as you help yourself heal from shin splints. A couple of times a week will not be enough. And try not to hurry. You must hold a stretch for it to work, and you might find yourself becoming a bit bored. Practice patience. And above all, be gentle when stretching. If it hurts, back off. If a stretch goes no further without discomfort, don't force the stretch past that point. Ever. Be gentle and you won't injure yourself while stretching.

How long should you hold a stretch? Over the years I've heard figures from two seconds all the way up to sixty seconds, and a wide variety within that range. Basically, they've all worked for me. As long as I did the stretches in the first place, and didn't get too rough while doing them. I've listed the very general estimate in this book of holding a stretch 10-20 seconds, then repeating that stretch three or four times. Why? It's worked for the masses over time, and is a good general rule of thumb. If you find holding a stretch shorter or longer than 10-20 seconds works better, then do it that way. Experiment and find the best duration of stretching for you personally.

You're encouraged to do all described stretches for both left and right sides, even if you are only suffering a shin issue on one side. All of the motions help to prevent injury as well as relieve existing soreness, so it's recommended to establish flexibility on both your left and right.

Muscle tightness contributes to shin splints, and we want to rectify that inflexibility as much as possible. Just remember to be consistent, patient, and gentle, and your stretching endeavor will be effective.

Stretch Your Shin Muscles

The stretches described in this section all stretch the anterior tibialis. The posterior tibialis is stretched as part of the calf stretches, discussed in the next section.

Seated Shin Stretch

This shin stretch is very simple yet quite effective, and it can be performed most anywhere. Use a gentle touch and very little force at all times with this motion. Excessive force here could be rough on your shin, but might especially endanger your ankle joint. You naturally don't need additional worries on top of having shin splints; go easy. That said, let's proceed with the left shin.

To begin, while sitting in a chair or on a bench, keep your right foot on the floor and cross the left leg over to the right leg, so that your left ankle rests on your right thigh. Place the fingers of your right hand on top of your left foot's toes, and the thumb of that hand along the ball of the left foot. Then gently bend the foot towards you (see Figure 5).

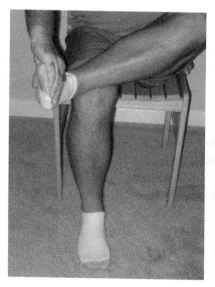 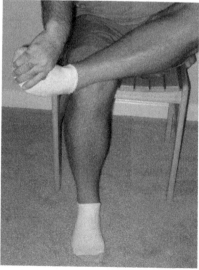

Figure 5: Seated shin stretch for your left shin starting position (left picture) and stretched position (right picture).

As you bend the foot towards yourself – and this next part is crucial for the shin stretch – slightly torque the toes towards the ceiling. This should impart the start of a twist. As you pull gently up and initiate the very start of that twist, you should feel a subtle stretch along the muscles in the front of your shin, the anterior tibialis. If you don't include the soft twisting motion, very little stretching will occur in your shin.

If you are in the early throes of the shin splints ordeal, don't expect to bend your foot very far before you feel some soreness. Stop the stretch if you feel pain at any point. Ease up, and stretch your shin muscle to a lesser degree. If you attempt to stretch the area further than it's ready to be stretched, you could injure yourself further. Developing flexibility anywhere in the body is a gradual process, and nowhere is this truer than in the often tight muscles of the shin.

Hold the Seated Shin Stretch for about 10-20 seconds, and repeat the process three or four times. Then reverse directions and perform the stretch for your other side.

Dragging Shin Stretch

Here's another movement done to encourage flexibility in the front of the shin. The stretch works, is convenient, and it's likely a stretch you've never tried before. At least not purposely!

The move is called the Dragging Shin Stretch, because, well, the movement is pretty much done by dragging your foot behind you. It will target the front of the shin, and while providing significant relief there, the Dragging Shin Stretch also assists in flexibility of the ankle.

To perform the stretch, stand with your hands on a counter, chair, or against a wall to steady yourself. The surface of the floor won't matter, whether it's a gym floor or one at home covered with tile or carpet. Also, you can do this stretch with shoes on or barefoot.

We'll stretch the right leg first in this case. Start with your feet together. Take a step forward with your left leg and put your bodyweight squarely on that foot. Rotate your right foot so that the tops of your right toes are touching the ground (see Figure 6).

To then activate the stretch, bend your left knee very slightly, lower your right knee toward the floor, and slowly drag the toes of the right foot forward on the ground. Keep your toes in firm contact with the floor so there's resistance against the foot's movement as you impart the forward pulling motion. Also make sure to keep the left knee just slightly bent, never extending it over the front of your left foot's toes; this is to prevent undue strain on your left knee.

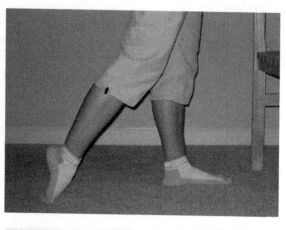

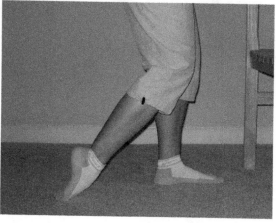

Figure 6: Dragging shin stretch for your right shin starting position (top picture) and stretching position (bottom picture).

You should feel a stretch from the ankle and top of your right foot through the front of your shins. Once you feel the stretch take effect, go no further and hold it at that point for 10-20 seconds. Rest a moment, and repeat three or four times. Then reverse directions and perform the stretch for your other leg.

Stair Shin Stretch

Here's another nice stretch for loosening up and protecting your shins' anterior tibialis muscles. It is a very easy motion as well. Let's start with the left leg.

Stand on a flight of stairs and shift your weight onto your right foot. Place your left heel at the edge of the step (see Figure 7). Then lower the toes of your left foot, while keeping your heel firmly in place. Only go as far as is comfortable; do not overextend and injure the muscle.

As you do the downward motion with your toes, the stretching action will take place in the front of your shins. That's all there is to it. Once you feel the stretch take effect, go no further and hold it at that point for 10-20 seconds. Rest a moment, and repeat three or four times. Then switch legs and stretch your right shin muscles.

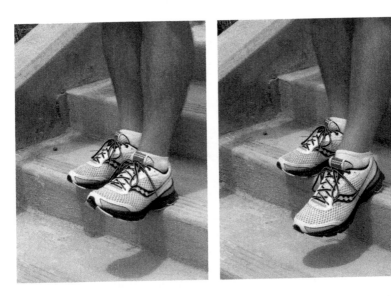

Figure 7: Stair shin stretch starting position (left picture) and stretched position (right picture).

Stretch Your Calf Muscles

Flexibility in your calf muscles is crucial to reducing the risk of injuries to your heels, feet, upper leg muscles, and also your shins; its importance cannot be overstated. The calf muscle works incredibly hard any time you walk or run; in the human body, only the heart muscle does more work than the calf. So lack of flexibility in the calf will cause unwelcome wear on your body day after day. Limberness in this area is vital to recovery from shin splints.

The repetitive impact from motions like running and walking eventually causes your related muscles and tendons to become short and tight. This is already hard on the shins, and a tight calf area stresses it even more. Tight calves will cause the muscles on the front of your lower leg to struggle as they flex your foot and ankle. This will continue to aggravate already ailing shins.

Tight calf muscles can cause a chain reaction of stress up the entire leg, including the shins, exerting additional strain on it. While under this increased tension, the introduction of any of the other factors which contribute to shin splints (bad shoes, excessive exercise, muscle weakness, hazardous surfaces, etc.) exacerbates the damage. Already embattled with duress, the shins undergo extra strain and impact from tightness in the calf. Tight calf muscles interfere with normal foot and leg mechanics, and your shins suffer as a consequence. Making your calves more limber will reduce the strain on your shins.

Remember, once again: think gentle whenever stretching any region of the body, calves included; wrenching really hard on tight muscles can cause strains and tears. You don't want to end up with any new injuries. That said, if you engage in endurance sports or rigorous exercise, you might find yourself amazed at the reduction in tenderness and the return of durability your shin region will experience once flexibility in the calf area gets established. Our bodies are like one long chain, and many of the parts are interconnected. Dedicate yourself to the simple stretches that follow and realize big dividends.

Seated Calf Stretch

While sitting on a comfortable surface, extend both legs in front of you. Reach forward carefully and grab your toes and the balls of your feet. (You can bend your knees as necessary; the stretch still works with bent knees.) Ever so mildly, pull the top of your feet back toward you, to the point that you feel a stretch begin. You should feel the effect in your calf muscles. Pull no further; hold that position and let the stretch take place (see Figure 8).

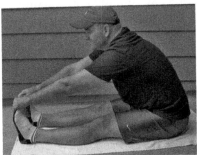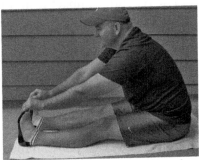

Figure 8: Seated calf stretch starting position (left picture) and stretched position (right picture).

If you presently have some difficulty reaching your feet in this position, as many people do, first wrap a towel around the bottom of your feet, then extend your legs in front of you (see Figure 9). With this extra reach in place, proceed with the calf stretch in the same way as described above. Position the towel around the balls of your feet, and initiate the stretch with a light touch. Once you feel the stretch take effect, stretch no further and hold it at that point.

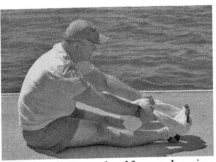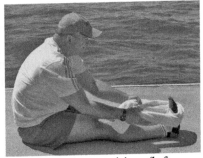

Figure 9: Seated calf stretch using a towel starting position (left picture) and stretched position (right picture).

Maintain the stretch for 15-20 seconds, and repeat the process three or four times.

Lunge Position Calf Stretch

This stretch shines due to both its effectiveness and its versatility. You won't need to don special exercise clothes or lie down on the floor. It can be done just about anywhere and at almost any time, regardless of what you're wearing. Furthermore, items like a dresser, a chair, or even a tree or a wall can be used to brace yourself as you conduct the stretch. The ready availability of the lunge position stretch makes it ideal to do while out on a walk, at work, or before and after any exercise session.

Place your hands on one of the stabilizing objects described above and the leg to be stretched set back behind you, foot flat on the ground. The front leg will be slightly bent at the knee. To execute the stretch, let your forward leg flex a bit more at the knee, and maneuver your hips slightly forward. Gently move into the stretch (see Figure 10). Once you feel the stretch in the calf area go no further and hold the stretch. Hold for 15-20 seconds. Repeat the sequence three or four times, and then switch legs.

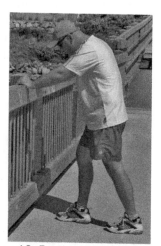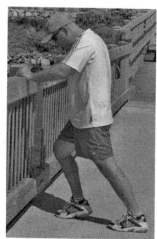

Figure 10: Lunge position stretch starting position (left picture) and stretched position (right picture).

Seated Arch Plus Stretch

In addition to stretching out your calf area to reduce strain on the shins, you can stretch the arch of the foot itself. This will help with optimal walking and running mechanics, reducing the pulling and strain experienced by the shins when the muscles below it are inflexible. (This is also a great stretch for foot health.)

The procedure for this stretch is as follows (let's start with the right leg): while sitting, set your right leg on your opposite knee. Grab your toes and the ball of your foot, and gently bend the foot back (see Figure 11). Hold the stretch for about 10-20 seconds, and repeat the process three or four times. Switch to your other leg.

Stop the stretch if you feel pain at any point. Ease up, and stretch your arch and calf to a lesser degree. If you attempt to stretch the area further than it's ready to be stretched, you could injure yourself further. Developing flexibility anywhere in the body is a gradual process, and nowhere is this truer than in the arch. Once the arch achieves extra flexibility, though, you'll undergo less harmful torque throughout the entire lower leg, including the shin.

I recommend doing this stretch a little later in the morning instead of first thing upon awakening. All parts of your body will be stiffened from sleep, especially your arch. You may want to move around for a while and then do the arch stretch. Your foot, ankle, and heel area will then be warmed up from stepping and walking, and may be more safely stretched. If you do decide to stretch your arches early in the morning, before walking, do so with extra care. Slow motion and ultra-gentle would be the idea in that case.

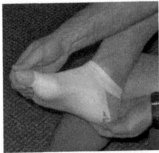 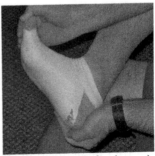

Figure 11: Arch Plus stretch starting position (left picture) and stretched position (right picture).

Stretch Your Upper Legs

Tightness in the upper leg muscles can place additional strain on the shin area when walking and running. Here you'll find a handful of simple motions to improve that situation.

A lack of flexibility in your quadriceps can impair a healthy walking and running gait, and the duress traveling down your kinetic chain can stress the shins more than necessary as you struggle to move along.

In a similar way, tight hamstrings can be tough to live with. Not only do inflexible hamstrings put these long, strong muscles in the back of your thighs themselves at risk, but they also cause undue tension on other body parts. The most publicized by-product of stiff hamstrings is the extra wear and tear they cause on the lower back. Similarly, tight hamstrings place extra stress on the shins.

It's a somewhat complex series of events. Lack of hamstring flexibility can cause less-than-ideal leg motions. One example is over-flexion of the knee. When the knee over-flexes, the effect travels down the leg, and excess flexion of the ankle increases as well. This then exerts extra stress on the shins; this can contribute to shin splints occurring and sticking around.

In addition, flexible and strong quadriceps and hamstring muscles assist in dissipating the force that travels throughout the leg when walking or running. When they're overly tight, neither set of muscles can do their part in this impact reduction. Simply put, inflexible quadriceps and hamstrings are quite taxing on other body parts, including the shins. Allowing them to stay inflexible means the progress in your shin splint recovery will be hindered.

We'll begin with the hamstrings. A number of good hamstring stretches are out there, and here's one that is effective, safe, and somewhat relaxing.

Supine Hamstring Stretch

While on your back, raise one leg, keeping it bent at the knee just a bit, hold the leg behind the knee, and slowly, gently extend that leg (see Figure 12). This will stretch the hamstring area. Expect the hamstring to be a little tight if you have not stretched it regularly.

A slight variation to this procedure is to wrap a towel around the center of your foot, versus holding your leg with your hands. Pull carefully on the towel as you extend your leg, stopping and holding the position once you feel a stretch begin.

Hold the stretch for about 10-20 seconds, and repeat the process three or four times. Switch to your other leg and repeat.

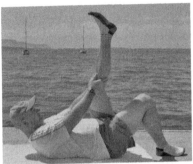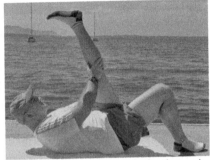

Figure 12: Supine hamstring stretch starting position (left picture) and stretched position (right picture).

Of all the endeavors listed in this book, developing hamstring flexibility is one of the most beneficial to your entire body. It assists in ease of movement in just about every motion your body can perform, in both your exercise routine and your daily tasks. And it feels good, almost a relief, when tight hamstrings get good and loosened up.

Quadriceps Stretch

Like tight hamstrings, inflexible quadriceps muscles can cause extra torque and a resulting strain on other body parts, such as the knees, lower back, and the shin area. This can happen especially if you run. Besides exposing you to less risk of an overuse injury, once you loosen up your quadriceps muscles a little, your legs will perform with more efficiency and power.

Try the following simple motion to increase your quadriceps flexibility. Use a table, chair, or counter to keep your balance. Bend your left leg up behind you, and grasp that foot with your left hand. Lift your heel towards your butt, while keeping your knees together and your back straight (see Figure 13). Raise your foot up until you feel a stretch in the front of your thigh. Hold the stretch for 10-20 seconds. Rest a moment, and repeat.

Then grasp your right leg with your right hand and do the stretch with your right leg. Hold the stretch for about 10-20 seconds, and repeat the process three or four times.

(Note: this motion is especially valuable as it does double-duty, giving you a gentle stretch in the front of your shin as well as your quadriceps area.)

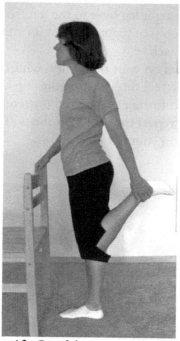

Figure 13: Quadriceps stretch (left leg).

Seated Ankle-on-Thigh Hip Flexor Stretch

Extra tight hips can throw off your gait and hinder a healthy stride. The stress can ultimately carry over to wear and tear on the shins, so we want to work on flexibility in the hip area.

Here is another stretch that can be performed most anywhere. This hip stretch is very simple yet quite effective. It's simple to explain as well.

To begin, sit down in the chair of your choice, or a bench, step, or the floor for that matter. The exact seat you choose won't make a difference. Cross the right leg over to the left, so that your right ankle rests on your left thigh (see Figure 14). Sit up straight; it won't work properly if you lean back.

Gently push down on your right knee, while gently lifting up your right ankle. Once you feel the areas of your hip and outside thigh start to stretch, go no further and hold the stretch for 10-20 seconds. Rest a moment, and repeat three or four times. Then switch legs to perform the stretch on your left leg.

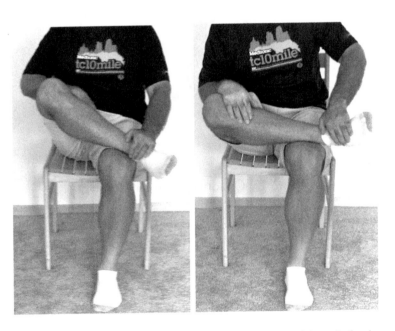

Figure 14: Seated ankle-on-thigh stretch starting position (left picture) and stretching position (right picture).

Strengthen Your Lower Legs

Next we'll work on some strength building, as it will add to your durability and enhance healing. In the exercises that follow, there will be a focus on the primary muscles in your shins, such as those that move your foot away from your shin (plantar flexion), those that move it towards your shin (dorsiflexion), and those muscles which are involved in lateral ankle motions, rotary ankle motions, and foot stabilization.

Some of the following strengthening motions are obvious, as they work directly on your lower leg muscles. Other suggested exercises focus on regions many people might not suspect as being related to shin stability. These non-shin muscle groups may not be as apparent, but they too are important for shin splint prevention and recuperation, as they're involved in the entire kinetic chain of the body's stability and mobility system.

For example, some important muscles for shin splint prevention that happen to be far above the shin are those of your butt, the gluteal muscles. Hardly an obvious piece of the shin splint puzzle, right? But the gluteus muscle group holds your pelvis upright and in a stable position as you stand, walk, and run. If your gluteus muscles, especially the gluteus medius, are not strong enough to provide this stabilization and align the femur, knee, and ankle, you are likely to overpronate your feet. As stated earlier, overpronation can contribute to shin splint development. So this area of important muscles, among others, will be addressed in this section.

Let's take a look.

Gentle Dorsiflexion

This is an exercise involving *dorsiflexion*, the important shin and foot action that primarily involves moving the toes closer to the shin. The motion uses a number of muscles of the lower leg, the main one being the all-important tibialis anterior.

Here we're going to purposely work those tibialis anterior muscles, building some extra endurance and strength to enhance your shin recuperation process. The exercise is simple to do and it works.

While sitting, keep your knees bent, your legs relaxed, and your heels on the ground. Then just bend your feet upwards, and flex your toes toward your shin (dorsiflexion). Once fully flexed, hold that position for a few seconds (see Figure 15). Then lower your feet and rest your toes back on the ground. Rest for a few seconds, then repeat. You have the option of doing both legs at once, as shown in Figure 15, or you can do one leg at a time. Or you can even alternate. Do whichever you're most comfortable with.

Complete the flexion about 12-15 times, or until the motion gets difficult and you can only do another repetition or two. Once you get to that point, you're done for now with this exercise. One set is enough when starting out with this strengthener. Do this sequence every other day.

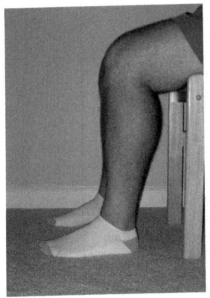 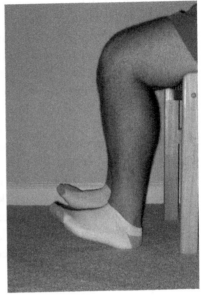

Figure 15: Gentle dorsiflexion starting position (left picture) and flexing position (right picture).

After you've performed a given motion on a few different days, you can add another set. I list the general, all-purpose approximation of 12-15 reps, but the optimal repetition total will vary from person to person, depending on that individual's current strength. I also state that instead of the ballpark figure of 12-15 reps, you can do the exercise until the motion simply gets difficult and you can only do another repetition or two. Once you hit that point, stop. That set is now done; move on. Your total reps may be only three or four, or may be 30 or 40. Again, it all depends on the strength you have when starting out.

As your strength improves, you can gradually increase the total repetitions. If any exercise here causes pain, cease doing it. A slight "burn" in the muscle is fine, but sharp pain is not. You may need to rest another week or two until you're ready for a particular motion.

Resisted Dorsiflexion

Once again we'll work the tibialis anterior muscle with a dorsiflexion motion. This time, however, we'll add some resistance to it.

Dorsiflexion always involves the motion of bringing the toes closer to the shin. In the Resisted Dorsiflexion exercise that will still be the goal, but in this case you'll make your shin muscles work harder to do so. Adding this resistance will thus accelerate your strength gains in that area.

There are some other methods out there for performing dorsiflexion with resistance, such as those involving ankle weights, rubber bands, and weight training machines. Those are all good ways to carry out this strengthening motion. In this scenario, however, we'll provide all the resistance your shins should need exclusively with your own body. You'll be doing an isometric exercise here, letting your muscles work against a nearly immovable object, which is a classic and proven method to improve strength and stability.

To begin, take a seat on the floor; on a carpet or mat is ideal. We'll start with your left leg as the exerciser. Keep that leg out, relaxed and relatively straight in front of you. Point the left foot's toes away from you. Place your right foot over the left one (see Figure 16). (It works best if your right foot "toes in" at this point, versus "toeing out.")

Now put a little pressure on the left foot with your right foot, and at the same time start to flex the left foot's toes closer to that shin. Exert enough force with the right leg so the left foot is unable to get to a full dorsiflexion position. Let those muscles struggle and work against the stronger force of the "blocking" foot. Stop the dorsiflexion at the halfway point, and hold the isometric exertion for a few seconds. Then relax it and rest for 10 seconds or so. Repeat the resisted flexions two or three more times, holding the halfway position, or maybe a little less than halfway or a bit past that point.

This will let the muscles get a good flexion workout in various phases of dorsiflexion.

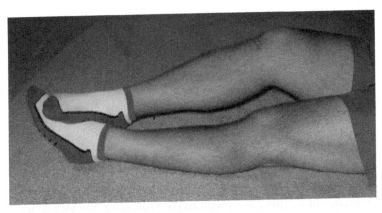

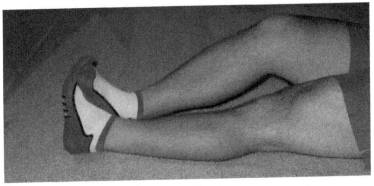

Figure 16: Resisted dorsiflexion starting position (top picture) and flexing position (bottom picture).

Don't worry that you won't be able to provide adequate resistance in this way; your right leg can easily overpower the left in this situation, as the right leg's quadriceps, rump, and hip muscles are all working against the other's much smaller shin and ankle muscles. It makes for strong resistance and a great way to tax and build up the targeted shin muscles.

Complete the exertion three or four times total, for just a few seconds each time. Then switch legs and do it the other way, letting the right shin work against the left leg and foot.

You can also try this movement while sitting in a chair; that works as well, but you might find it less awkward to simply sit on the floor instead.

Do the Resisted Dorsiflexion exercise every other day.

Heel Walking

For this exercise, we'll include some mobility while giving your shin muscles a workout.

With your foot in a dorsiflexed position (the front of your foot pulled up towards your shin), walk around on your heel for a few steps (see Figure 17, left picture). Keep your foot dorsiflexed throughout this drill. Don't let your toes touch the ground. After a few days of repeating the exercise and getting the feel for it, walk the entire length of the room a time or two, or take it outside and see how far you can go.

Make sure to perform this strengthening motion slowly and under control: no speed or bouncing needed.

You can perform this exercise one heel at a time or with both feet in the dorsiflexed position. If doing both heels at the same time (as shown in the right picture of Figure 17) and balance is an issue, walk along a wall or railing which you can use for support. You'll find that in order to keep your toes in the dorsiflexed position, your stride will shorten.

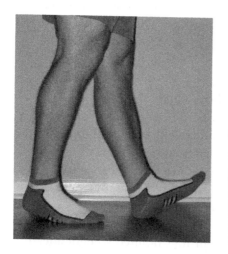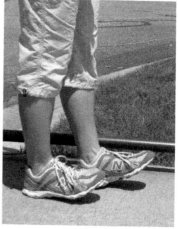

Figure 17: Heel walking to strengthen the shin muscles: one heel (left picture), and both heels (right picture).

Do this motion for just a couple of minutes, every other day, as you recover. After three or four days of repeating the heel walking, push yourself a little and do it until you can feel the first signs of muscle exhaustion or a slight "burn" setting in. Then call it a workout, and give the motion a rest for a day. The day after that, repeat it.

Toe Walking

In this next exercise, mobility will also be put into play, and this time the workout is focused on the rear of the lower leg, the calf and soleus muscles.

With your feet in a plantar flexed position (in other words, up on the toes and the balls of your feet), walk around as you did in the previous exercise, while up on your heels. Keep your foot plantar flexed throughout this exercise. Don't let your heels touch the ground. After a few days of repeating the motion and getting the feel for it, walk the entire length of the room a time or two.

Make sure to perform this strengthening motion at a slow, deliberate pace; avoid any fast or frantic movement. Do the Toe Walking routine for just a couple of minutes, every other day, as you recover. After three or four days of repeating this toe walking maneuver, feel free to go a little longer than you did at first, until it's clear the calf and soleus muscles are tiring. Then end this strengthener and rest it for a day. The day after that, repeat the exercise.

The Alphabet Drill and Toe Taps

Here are two closely related and equally beneficial motions to build strength and endurance in your shin muscles.

The Alphabet Drill is a simple but effective exercise for strengthening all of your lower leg muscles. This movement is easy to perform and can be done most anywhere.

To begin, simply sit in a chair or on a bench and hold one foot suspended above the floor with your toes pointed straight ahead. Then trace all of the letters of the alphabet with your toes. This simple exercise will use nearly every muscle in your lower leg. One time through the alphabet is usually enough. Switch legs and repeat on the other foot.

Toe Taps are even easier: you don't even have to know the alphabet. (Grin.) To perform this exercise, again just sit in a chair or on a bench, with your feet resting on the floor. Then use the front of your foot to tap the floor while keeping your heel anchored. Just do this tapping motion for a minute or so. Eventually work up to two or three minutes of steady tapping. You can do one foot at a time, or both feet at once.

A few bouts of the Alphabet Drill combined with some sessions of Toe Taps make for leisurely – and often amusing – workouts. But be confident in the fact that actual conditioning of your lower legs is taking place, and that these motions are contributing to recovery and prevention of shin pain. Be sure to make the two drills part of your routine, and do them every other day.

Calf Raises

You got some calf strengthening with the Toe Walking described earlier; we want to continue on with that effort, since calf stability is so crucial to shin splint prevention and recovery. To help stabilize the motion of your lower legs, ankles, and feet, you'll want to focus on building strength in your calf muscles. Strong muscles in your calf area assist in controlling the action of the foot's strike, roll, and push-off with each step. The stronger your calves are, the more your feet will be stabilized during this process, and consequently the less strain your shins will experience.

Strengthening your calf muscles will deliver the extra benefit of greater endurance: you'll be able to work, exercise and stand in place longer without tiring your lower legs. Your shins in turn will receive better support and protection. This will make things like doing endurance training, getting through a workday on your feet, and having fun outdoors more attainable.

Your calves get worked during just about any movement you make on your feet or with your legs. Walking, biking, running, playing tennis, and climbing stairs are just a few examples of activities which involve your calf muscles, as well as many other muscles simultaneously. To isolate the calves and work just them primarily, you can use the following simple yet effective exercise.

While standing, hold onto a railing, table, or the back of a chair for balance. Then, raise yourself up so your heels leave the ground, and you balance on the balls of your feet. Lower your heels back down, and you have just completed one repetition (see Figure 19).

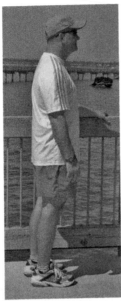 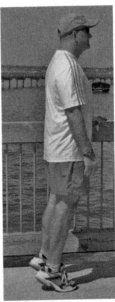

Figure 19: Standing calf raise starting position (left picture) and flexed position (right picture).

Continue with the exercise until your calf muscles start to feel some exhaustion. Then stop to rest. That is one set. The capacity for the calves to perform isolated strength training like this varies greatly from person to person. For you, this may range from 5 repetitions up to 35, or maybe more. Just complete one set while getting used to this routine early on. After a couple of weeks of doing the exercise, add a second set. Do these every other day as you recover from the shin splint injury. Once you work back into walking and running as you did previously, only do calf raises once a week at the most to avoid overtraining.

Once you build up adequate strength, you can perform the exercise while holding a pair of dumbbells to provide greater resistance. Or, just do more repetitions. Either way builds both strength and endurance; a routine with more weight and less repetitions sides toward strength building, less weight with more repetitions emphasizes endurance. Both are beneficial.

Towel Scrunch

Just as stronger lower leg muscles help you heal from shin splints sooner, so too will a stronger arch in your foot. A powerful arch will smooth your foot's landing, assist in a good push-off, and help the foot absorb impact.

Fortunately, developing strength in the arch of your foot is not hard. Sometimes, it's actually kind of fun. You just have to make a habit of it. See the following exercise for some easy yet valuable arch strengthening. This exercise also works your shin muscles, so you're getting a nice two-for-one here. Do this motion while seated in a comfortable chair.

Place a towel on the floor in front of you. Use just your toes to drag or "scrunch" the towel toward you (see Figure 18). You should be able to feel the muscles in your arch really flex. Success is attained when you've scrunched the entire towel into a bunch. Repeat the action again. Do this every other day, and try to work up to about 8 or 10 repetitions over time. (Note: you'll find it easier to do the towel scrunch on a smooth surface; carpet can impart excessive resistance when using a terry cloth towel.)

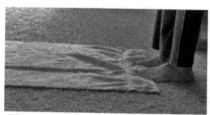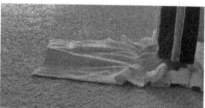

Figure 18: Towel scrunch starting position (left picture) and during the scrunching (right picture).

Strengthen Your Hips

As stated earlier, a lack of hip and pelvic stability can cause an increased load to be exerted upon the shins, especially if you're a runner. Here is a group of easy hip and pelvic stabilizing motions that will make your gait more stable and cause less strain to be ultimately endured by your shin area.

The *gluteus medius*, an all-important muscle for shin stability and health, is crucial in controlling the level of the hips. Weakness in the gluteus medius can result in an abnormal gait cycle where the hip of the swinging leg drops down, rather than raises up. This results in excess knee flexion in order for the foot to clear the ground. Over time, this can cause overuse injuries, one of the main ones being shin splints. So let's strengthen that gluteus medius area.

If any exercise here causes pain, cease doing it. A slight "burn" in the muscle is fine, but sharp pain is not. You may need to rest another week or two until you're ready for a particular motion.

Lying Hip Abduction

Begin this important strengthening exercise lying on your left side. Propping your head up on your elbow is fine, as is resting your head on a pillow. Brace yourself by placing your right hand on the floor in front of you. Extend both legs to a straight position, keeping your entire body in a straight line (see Figure 20). For added stability, you may also bend the lower leg back at the knee.

Keep your back, hips, and knees straight and facing forward. Slowly lift your upper leg straight up towards the ceiling, tightening the muscles at the side of your hip: the gluteus medius.

Make sure to keep your pelvis in place, facing forward. Raise the leg up as high as possible, hold it at the top for a second, then slowly lower the leg back down. Repeat about 12-15 times, or until the motion gets difficult and you can only do another repetition or two. Flip onto your other side and perform the exercise with the left leg.

As your gluteal strength improves, you can gradually increase the total repetitions, or add an additional set of 12-15 repetitions. Do this exercise every other day.

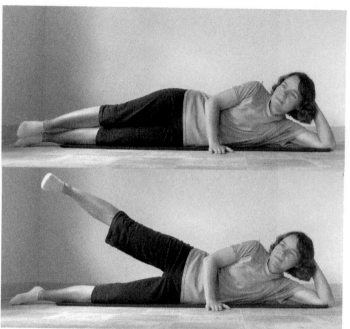

Figure 20: Lying hip abduction (right leg) starting position (top picture) and flexed position (bottom picture).

Lying Hip Abduction with Dumbbell

Here you'll add a little weight resistance to the hip abduction motion, in order to increase the load and build strength. If you do this exercise with shorts on, you may want to use a rubber-coated dumbbell to protect your skin. If you have no dumbbells, you could use a weight plate, or even something like a big, fat phonebook for additional resistance.

Lie on your side on the floor or on a mat (see Figure 21). Extend the top leg to a straight position, with the lower leg bent back at the knee underneath for stability. Grasping a dumbbell or weight with your top hand, position the dumbbell as close to the knee as possible on the top side of your thigh facing the ceiling. Make sure to keep your pelvis facing forward.

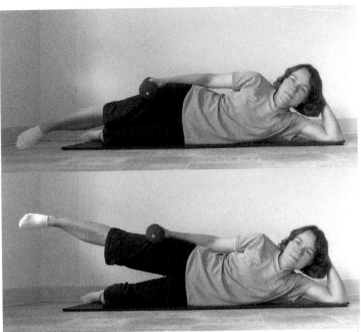

Figure 21: Lying hip abduction with dumbbell starting position (top picture) and flexed position (bottom picture), working the right leg.

Raise the weighted leg up as high as possible, keeping the dumbbell positioned on the side of the upper thigh. Return the leg to the floor and repeat. Repeat about 12-15 times, or until the motion gets difficult and you can only do another repetition or two, whichever comes first. Then flip onto your other side and perform the exercise with the opposite leg.

Again, as your gluteal strength improves, you can gradually increase the total repetitions to a point where you feel fatigue in the muscle, or instead add an additional set of 12-15 repetitions. Do this exercise every other day.

Side Plank

Also referred to as the *side bridge,* the side plank can be an essential tool for developing solid hip abductors, as well as stability in the pelvis, spine, and hips. Again, strength in these areas will help you fend off and heal from shin splints.

Lie on your left side, propping yourself up on your forearm. Keep your elbow directly below your shoulder. Your legs should be straight and your ankles together. Push your hips off the ground by engaging your hip and abdominal muscles until your body is in a straight line (see Figure 22); brace yourself with your forearm. Ensure your head is in line with your neutral spine. See if you can hold the position for 10 seconds or so. If 10 seconds becomes easy, go for 20. Flip onto your other side and repeat.

Once you've held the position for the target duration, give the motion a rest until next time. Do this exercise every other day.

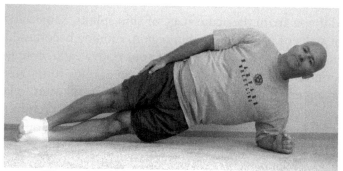

Figure 22: Side plank working the left side.

Important tips: Keep your abdominals tight while performing the side plank, and do not let your hips sag to the floor. Also, your head and neck should be in line with your spine.

Other Strengtheners

Grinding out repetitions with focused exercises brings undeniably positive results, but they are not the only way to improve your durability. Part of an effective active recovery plan includes activities that keep you on the move in order to maintain endurance, add strength, and hopefully provide you with a pleasant experience. Here are some more activities to consider as your shins heal.

Keep Moving: Bike for Exercise

Unless you are already a triathlete, you may find yourself in a quandary regarding exercise due to your shin splint ordeal. Perhaps you were in the good habit of walking for exercise, and that routine has now been tripped up by your injury. Even walking on a treadmill might hurt, despite its built-in cushion. Or if you like to hike, this reality of tenderness is even more true, given the steep nature and unpredictable texture of many trails.

And if you are in the acute stage of shin splints, subjected to frequent stabs of pain in your shin region, running becomes highly questionable. The pounding down of your bodyweight, coupled with the sheer number of footfalls realized on an average run, translates into a taxing experience for your injury. Yet you still want to keep moving, stay strong, and burn some calories. You may return to walking, hiking, and yes, even running in due time. But for now you need an alternative aerobic exercise source. What to do?

Consider biking.

Biking is a great cardiovascular workout. It is a non-weight bearing exercise, so stress and jarring on your shins area will be minimal. In addition, biking will provide incredible quadriceps conditioning. Your hamstrings, buttocks, hips, and calves will get in on the action too. It will help you improve endurance and strength, and add to the muscle mass in your legs and lower body. And with any gain in solid body mass, you will burn more energy even while resting. This quiet sizzle of calories will help you maintain your fitness. And any weight gain you can stave off will mean that much less force on your legs, helping to speed your recovery.

You can ride a bike with intensity, but for moderate aerobic and strength training, feel free to ride casually. You'll still get plenty of exercise. As a matter of fact, once you slow way down, the resistance experienced to get back up to speed will be greater than if you were going fast, since you've lost forward momentum. The aerobic training and strength development will be substantial, and so will the energy you burn for weight control.

To protect your body, observe a couple of technique tips when biking. Make sure your knees go pretty much straight up and down; don't angle them outwards, away from the bike. The straight up and down motion will exert less strain on your lower legs as well as your knees. Also, push the pedals with the middle of the foot, not the ball of the foot. The mechanics of pushing with the ball of the foot can stress injured shins. Pumping the pedals with the midfoot, on the other hand, will exert little strain there.

Of course, any benefits realized by riding a bike with wheels can also be attained by riding a stationary bike. In most ways, your body won't know the difference. Jump on either type of bike and move those pedals. It'll help you build endurance and some key leg muscles while avoiding inactivity.

Keep Moving: Walk This Way

To remain active, relieve stress, burn calories, and hasten your shin recovery, do some walking. Walking is a readily available, versatile, convenient, and inexpensive activity. It gives some folks peace of mind and as a result helps them improve their mood, stay positive, and even sleep better. And for such a seemingly gentle endeavor, it's quite effective in delivering results in terms of a workout.

If you are a runner, this section could be titled "Walk Instead of Run for Exercise." While in shin splint recovery mode, you may want to avoid the high impact of running, and walk instead. Walking can greatly assist in some serious conditioning and strengthening of the lower leg, ankle, and foot areas, while subjecting you to very little impact.

To help your injury recovery as you perform your walking outings, try this approach to walking. First of all, shorten your stride. You might want to seize the moment and make your walks into a vigorous workout, and thus reach way out with each leg as you bounce up and down, lunging forward to conquer as much distance as you can with each stride. Don't.

A real long stride is hard on your body in general, and can be quite detrimental to the lower leg while it's healing. Instead, keep your stride short. If you want to cover more ground in less time, just take quicker steps.

Next, adjust your foot placement with each landing so you land with your midfoot. Hitting hard on the back of the heel can stress the shins. And don't walk on the balls of your feet or your toes. While that's okay for a short-term strengthening session as described in the Toe Walking section, actually walking this way is detrimental for your lower legs. Simply set down each foot while making most of the contact with the front of your heel, or the very middle of your foot. This will result in less wear and tear, and make your walking propulsion more efficient in general.

Last, keep your lower legs at ease and relaxed as you perform your stride. If you relax your lower legs, you'll eliminate lots of strain while you walk, largely because you'll reduce excess dorsiflexion of the foot (in other words, where your toes move closer to your shin). Among other things, excess dorsiflexion strains the tibialis anterior muscle on the front of the shins.

So for best results, walk along in an easygoing manner. Avoid the stiff and assertive "stalking" gait so many exercise enthusiasts take on, as they move along with a serious game face, smack their feet down with each step, and spring forward with aggression, demonstrating that they're on a mission. (You know you've seen this!) Instead, take it easy and allow your entire lower leg to move forward with a supple looseness as you step.

A relaxed stride with good foot placement will not only reduce excess dorsiflexion, it will minimize impact even further. The lack of impact realized while walking can be a huge plus. As you walk, the force exerted upon your feet is only about one and a half times your body weight. While running, by comparison, your feet often endure up to ten times this amount.

The payoff in terms of calorie burn and conditioning gained while walking fast are undeniable, but you don't have to speed walk or race walk. In fact, when you walk slowly, momentum doesn't continue to carry you forward as it does when you walk very fast, so your muscles work a bit more to lift and propel you from a near dead stop. In truth, slow, medium, and brisk walking speeds will all provide a good workout. Walk at the speed with which you're most comfortable. And if you ever find yourself becoming out of breath, slow down. You just don't have to push yourself that hard to reap the benefits of walking.

Even though walking is relatively easy on your shin area, increase the distance you walk gradually. You may feel gung ho about your walking program, ready to exceed past distances, explore new places, and burn even more calories. This type of enthusiasm is a great thing, but use common sense at the same time. Walking will not stress your shins like running, rugged hiking, or the fast stops and starts experienced in many sports. But it is still serious exercise. Walking will tax your muscles and connective tissue, which is actually one reason it's beneficial to you. It can be overdone, however, especially when shin splints are in their early stages. If a given distance results in increased pain, versus simple muscle soreness, cut back on the length of your walk for the time being. If your shin splints are in the acute stage, where pain is often quite sharp, you can inflict upon your vulnerable lower legs additional damage by trying too much too soon. Resist that urge.

So if you read or hear something to the effect that a person should walk at least six days a week for thirty or forty minutes at a time minimum, take the advice with a grain of salt. You may or may not be ready for that type of exertion. Be enthused but cautious. Use a gradual approach. You'll work up to greater frequency and distance with time. I've read the suggested amount of 10% by which to increase your distance per week, but that's just a ballpark figure. You can lengthen your walks by even less than that each week and still make good progress. Or, if you find a walk location or routine you really like, don't feel pressure to increase the distance at all. Regular and consistent walks are far more important than long ones. That should be your priority for a walking program, not setting new records each week.

If you can only walk five or eight minutes at a time, due to time constraints or your level of injury, try to repeat these time increments a few times a day. The positive effects of walking can be realized in a cumulative sense. Five walking outings of five minutes each is roughly as beneficial as a contiguous twenty-five minute session. If short walks are all you can fit in to your day, take heart and keep at it.

To minimize any additional trauma your lower legs might experience as you make strides to get back in the game, see the "Maintain Low Impact Form" commentary in "Section 1: Protect and Defend." Remember, shin splint recovery is a tricky business.

You need to keep moving, but avoid doing too much at the same time. And just as importantly, make sure you walk in good, supportive shoes, covered earlier in greater detail.

With that said, make a conscious effort to walk more, and plan the outings according to the amount your recovering shins will allow. It will strengthen and tone your entire lower body, including those crucial muscles of the lower leg and foot. It may also help you sleep better, lift your spirits, and encourage you to stay committed to your overall recovery program. Include some variety, challenge yourself slowly but surely, and enjoy yourself.

Keep Moving: Swim for Exercise

If you want an exercise that subjects you to no impact, strengthens your entire body, and burns calories like crazy, go swimming. If you haven't done much swimming in recent years, it may be the perfect answer for a change of pace and a needed fitness boost. In most cases, injured shins will suffer no ill effects from the rigors of swimming, even though your system will be going through grueling workouts.

I certainly am no expert on swimming techniques or strokes. I cannot outline a swimming regimen for fitness, but I know from experience that even a very short session will intensely work out a person's muscles and cardiovascular system.

For a person who has not used it much for exercise, swimming involves intense fitness demands. Even if you are in good condition for activities like biking, walking, and running, a swim can tax your aerobic and anaerobic abilities like nothing else. Swimming is an activity all its own. And for such a high value strengthening and calorie-consuming activity, swimming is surprisingly easy on the joints.

If you don't know how to swim, or it's been a long time since you have, consider swimming lessons. This period of recuperation on which you have embarked can be a time to try new things, and swimming might be a good challenge to tackle. And while you learn, you'll build endurance and strength while shedding quite a few calories. Maybe it will turn into a life-long activity for you.

Closely related to swimming is *deep water running*, which simulates running on land while wearing a flotation device. I've not yet tried this, but many athletes and coaches swear by it as a method of cross-training and injury recovery. Consider looking into a deep water running class at a local university or community pool. It could serve you well as a workout and an alternative to swimming if you're looking to mix up your activities further. And like with swimming, your lower legs will suffer no impact whatsoever.

For a total body workout that spares your shins of any abuse, dive into the swimming routine and get some serious exercise.

Keep Moving: Use Caution on the Treadmill

Treadmills can be versatile, valuable devices for health, strength maintenance, and stamina building. Countless fitness enthusiasts, novice through expert, make use of the treadmill for exercise. You may have used a treadmill to one degree or another before shin splints set in. If you plan on continuing with treadmill workouts, or starting them up for that manner, be sure to take note.

Treadmill usage can be especially taxing on the shins, especially the tibialis anterior on the front of the lower leg. This is why: treadmills operate with a moving belt upon which you maneuver. The task involved in this maneuvering, namely of pushing off and taking each new step on a twirling belt, is more difficult for the body to accomplish than it may appear in the heat of a workout. And that difficulty is focused mostly on the tibialis anterior, and happens in conjunction with human motion such as walking and running having developed by propulsion on solid surfaces. Not a twirling belt.

Now, a number of benefits can be achieved from treadmill training, and treadmills do have a big plus over solid ground in that they absorb impact. That in most cases is huge, and a big vote in favor of the treadmill. But we're concerned with shin health and recuperation here, and the movement occurring while on a treadmill is stressful to the shin muscles. There's no way around it.

If you continue to use a treadmill regardless, here's a tip: increase the incline and go slower. The steeper incline will increase the exertion of the workout in general, so you won't be taking the easy way out. But be reasonable in the level of incline you choose; setting it at the maximum can put too much strain on your lower leg muscles. So pay attention to what your body is telling you and adjust the incline to a level that doesn't add undue strain to your healing legs. (Note: nothing but uphill or "up-incline" can be tough on your

Achilles tendons as well; this can be minimized by taking very small steps as you run or walk on the treadmill.)

For reasons of shin muscle duress, if you're trying to recover from a case of shin splints, minimize your use of a treadmill. If you do choose to use a treadmill, set the incline higher, move slower with shorter steps, and go to it.

Section 3:
Nurture

Create the best possible healing atmosphere that you can for your injury. Your body wants to heal; help it along.

Stay Well-Hydrated

Hydration is often overlooked as a major factor in injury recovery. But replenishing your body with plenty of water and other nutritious fluids will give your shin splint recuperation a boost. Staying well-hydrated is very important to your overall health; if you're chronically dehydrated, shin splints may represent just one of your worries.

Maintaining ideal hydration benefits your digestion, skin, hair, brain function, strength, and endurance. Adequate hydration will help ward off colds and flu. It will assist in heart health. If a person's hydration level drops even 5%, metabolism can slow as much as 30%. So any weight maintenance or weight loss efforts will be far easier with regular water intake (which in turn might help you heal from shin splints: lower body weight = less shin strain).

When you become dehydrated, so do your ligaments, muscles, and tendons. Connective tissue in the human body depends on water for elasticity and stability. Muscle function, including that of your leg and foot muscles, will be diminished with dehydration. This is exacerbated as your body's blood volume is reduced, which in turn limits the oxygen reaching the muscles. Muscle performance will further suffer. This means weakening, tightness, and possible cramping. More strain on your shins will result.

So make a conscious effort to consume plenty of fluids each day. And drink before you get thirsty. Under normal circumstances, with normal food intake, that fluid can be primarily water. Drink about 5-8 glasses of water a day. The water content in liquids like milk, orange juice, hot cocoa, and vegetable juice does count. Water contained in alcohol and in caffeinated drinks like cola and coffee do not, due to the diuretic effect these beverages have on the body.

Of course, it's best to do all things in moderation. When replacing lost fluids, there is no need to drink a gallon of water in a sitting. Try to rehydrate with the approximate amount of water you lost over time, whether through normal activities or through vigorous work or exercise. If you are exercising heavily or enduring hot weather, in either case sweating profusely, you may want to consume a commercial sport drink to replace potassium, sodium, and other electrolytes at the same time that you rehydrate. This option is more effective for rejuvenation than plain water when fluid loss has been great, as described above. And it will help you avoid a condition known as *hyponatremia*, defined by a dangerously low concentration of sodium in the blood.

Hyponatremia results when heavy water loss takes place, and the only replacement you take for it is water alone; especially a large amount of water, which can cause the level of bloodstream minerals to drop. When mineral levels in your blood are low, such as sodium, water in your bloodstream may move into your brain, where concentrations of sodium are higher. This process is the normal attempt of human physiology to even things out. In this case, however, it can be bad news. The pressure in your brain could increase, and at the very least cause dizziness. It can also cause twitches, stupor, seizures, unconsciousness, and brain damage. So use good judgment when drinking back lost liquids.

Don't worry, an extra glass of water will not cause hyponatremia. A few extra glasses of plain water consumed at once might though, if you're dehydrated. When seeking replenishment, include some nutritious foods along with water, especially those containing potassium and sodium. Or as mentioned, consume a commercial sport drink, which will be designed to replace the lost minerals.

In short, be sensible when rehydrating. But by all means, make sure you take the time and effort to do it. Plan ahead and have drinks on hand before, during and after exercise, workdays, and outings of any kind. Adequate hydration can serve as a substantial aid in your healing process.

Massage Your Injured Area

Consider using self-massage to accelerate your shin healing process. A gentle palpitation of the injured area using both thumbs may work wonders to expedite your healing journey.

Massage can be used to break up scar tissue and restore full motion of soft tissue. Years of clinical evidence supports the effectiveness of deep tissue massage to treat strains and sprains, including injuries like shin splints. As you apply tension with massage over your injured area, you may help break up adhesions and restore proper blood flow to the tissues; a faster rate of healing is often the result.

The muscles along the shin, like the calf, soleus, and tibialis anterior, are all really tough muscles. But at first, perform the massage carefully. You may be tempted to really dig your thumbs in, but go easy. Remember, you're kneading *injured* tissues. Therefore, a light touch is the order of the day. Very forceful pressure could worsen the condition, if the area is already inflamed.

Proponents of massage believe that it encourages healing by manipulating the tissue at hand, and in so doing promotes relaxation, better blood flow, and the elimination of waste products. And in the case of shin splints, massage can serve to break up scar tissue that is forming and allow the injured tissue to heal faster.

The actual technique for self-massaging your shin area is simple. Sit on the floor, or a chair, bench, or couch; then use both hands to ensconce your lower leg, near the region of soreness. Place both thumbs upon the intended area.

To begin the massage, simply push in a few times, then run the thumbs up and down the length of the muscle, imparting gentle pressure at first, then some medium-level pressure after you've massaged the area for a minute or two. This serves to break up scar tissue and expedite healing. Focus on the tibialis anterior in the front of the shin, along the tibia bone. Then progress to the back of the lower leg, and target the calf and soleus muscles there.

Do this for a few more minutes, and feel the result. If certain spots trigger sharp pain, discontinue the massage in that location, at least for the time being. You may benefit from the same action in the future, maybe in a few weeks once your healing has progressed. Or perhaps massage is not the best thing for your particular condition. You might have to experiment while being cautious.

You may, on the other hand, experience significant relief immediately. You'll have to feel the situation out, no pun intended. If gentle massage does give you immediate relief, do it regularly as part of your regimen. Once a day is not too often. This convenient procedure may do the trick to erase soreness, clear out waste products in the tissues of your shin area, and quicken your recovery. It may also diminish the return of pain as you resume activity. And sometimes it just feels good!

Roll with It

With a rolling pin, that is!

Needless to say, proceed very gently and very carefully here, making sure to avoid the tibia itself (it is one of the most exposed bones in your body, as anyone who has ever smacked his or her shin bone can attest). This is yet another way to massage your injured area, with a slightly different approach than a massage by hand. Like massaging your lower leg by hand, gliding a rolling pin over your stressed shin area can break up adhesions that may be forming on the traumatized tissue, and allows a more complete and rapid healing process to take place. Blood flow will be improved as well, further enhancing healing. The process will help to reduce inflammation as well as whisk away waste materials, further assisting your injury in a quicker repair. Plus, as it's an active massage method, a rolling pin massage is actually a small workout in and of itself.

Like with any other massage, it mostly feels good, but there can also be moments of discomfort as you put pressure on the shin tissues to help break up the unwanted adhesions. Work into the rolling pin massage motion slowly; while you can adjust to some soreness, stop the regimen if true pain occurs. Severely strained tissues may need more rest time before being worked over through a massage routine.

To proceed, it's easiest to perform a rolling pin massage if you sit. With a movement both slow and deliberate, just roll the pin from the top of your front shin muscle, the tibialis anterior, to the bottom of it near the ankle. The first pass-through will show the power of the rolling pin compared to bare hands. Go easy. Pause on any tight or sore spots, and spend extra time on muscle areas that seem to have a knot in them. A few minutes total on one leg should be enough. Repeat the process on your other shin.

Then progress to the back of the lower leg, and target the calf and soleus muscles in that region for a few minutes.

Instead of a rolling pin, you can of course use other rolling massagers such as a back roller and similar.

Elevate Your Lower Legs

Any chance you get to elevate your lower legs, do so. Elevating them will enhance blood flow and aid in the removal of waste products from the injury. Elevation reduces the blood pressure in the area and thus the swelling. Additionally, the improved circulation will allow better delivery of nutrients to the injured tissue, helping the tissue heal. Your recovery process will speed up as a result.

You basically want to elevate your lower legs above the level of your heart. Nothing too scientific here. The most practical way to do this is to simply lie on your back and prop your feet up. You can use a couple of pillows, or maybe even the couch or a cushioned chair.

Try to elevate the lower legs for 8-15 minutes. If you can only fit in 5 minutes or so at a given time, still treat yourself to it. Elevation of the lower legs is a course of action where you can feel the relief immediately. Especially if you've just been on your feet for a long time or you've been out walking or running. Once you do it a time or two, you'll probably need no further encouragement. Your shin area will feel noticeable relief. Not to mention, the session might give you a chance to unwind, read, or rest, so the benefits of powering down to prop up your lower legs may be multiple.

Whoever thought doing so little could do so much? Keep this effortless tactic in mind and use it to encourage your progress back to healthier shins. All while you lie down, stretch out, and relax.

Get Enough Sleep

Spend a little more time in bed and you might heal more quickly as a result. To expedite your recuperation from shin splints, it's in your interest to get plenty of sleep. It seems counterintuitive, but here's why it works.

During sleep your body takes many measures to restore itself; among these processes is the generation of Human Growth Hormone, a healing hormone your system naturally produces. During deep sleep, your body creates higher amounts of it.

In addition to helping you repair injuries, Human Growth Hormone enhances a slow, steady calorie burn; this helps regulate body fat and prevent excess weight gain in case you're forced to become inactive. Along the same line, Human Growth Hormone regulates your body's sensitive chemical balance, which helps control your appetite. So with no extra effort on your part, getting a good night's sleep allows you to manage your weight; sleep's weight control abilities can compensate for the fewer calories you may burn due to your being laid up.

Researchers have found that significant changes in the levels of the hormones ghrelin and leptin occur when you get less than 5 hours of sleep. After a few consecutive nights of poor sleep you may find yourself with an out-of-control appetite; this is mostly because sleep deprivation increases ghrelin and decreases leptin below normal levels. This sensitive hormone balance helps control your appetite. Ghrelin is used to whet your appetite; if its level is excessive, your appetite will be excessive as well.

Weight control and injury recovery aside, do you want to live sleep-deprived anyway? The inability to sleep can be a medical issue, and much more complex than we can completely discuss here. But many situations of sleep deprivation are caused by individual choices, like staying up late to surf the web, play video games, or, amazingly, watch late night TV programs even when sleepy. (Could these shows possibly be worth losing sleep over?)

Enough with my soap box moment. Here are some tips to acquire restorative sleep:

– Avoid caffeine a few hours before you plan to sleep. Old advice but still worth mentioning. Caffeine consumed eight or nine hours before you sleep will usually be cleared from your system before bedtime; caffeine consumed an hour or two before that time usually won't be.

— If you drink alcohol, pay attention to how it affects you and your sleeping experience. If you need to cut back, you'll know it. Then do it.

— If deep, sound sleep eludes you, keep in mind that lying still, in a neutral relaxed state, provides many of the same benefits as deep sleep. It can make for a long night just lying there waiting for sleep, but try to stay calm and simply rest. Above all, don't let anxiety about not sleeping ironically cause you to not sleep. Knowing the fact that calm rest is a close second to deep sleep can, interestingly enough, help you transition into sound sleep. That's been my experience.

— Read a book, paper, or magazine an hour or so before retiring, in place of using a computer or watching TV. The electronic media are believed to disturb normal sleep, in some cases and for some reason, whereas reading from print materials actually encourages preparation for sleep.

— If you get a chance to take a nap, do it. Not many of us have time for naps in today's sometimes-crazy world, but go for it if the opportunity arises.

    This thought has not been without controversy. In recent decades a few "experts" have proclaimed that naps are useless, and that they disrupt nighttime sleep. And, of all things, that they age you. Balderdash. If we weren't meant to take naps, and if the body and brain didn't yearn for them, we wouldn't take them. Treat yourself to a short nap when you can. It will encourage injury recovery.

— Go to sleep a little earlier if you can. Early birds wake up refreshed and seize the day, while night owls are the ones still walking around in a near zombie state at 9:00 AM, babbling about not being a morning person. For best results on your injury recuperation endeavor, you have to do what's best for your body and brain. Adequate sleep will be a big help in your recovery efforts. If for you that means going to sleep a little earlier, choose that option.

I believe this is a rare time that you'll see a firm recommendation to make sleep a priority for wound healing. Like adequate hydration, the need for a good night's sleep is often undervalued and overlooked when it comes to recovery from bodily injuries. For wound healing, trust me…better yet, trust science: adequate sleep can make a difference.

Consume Plenty of Antioxidants

For best results in the healing of just about any injury, you will want to decrease oxidative stress on your body. With that said, those diets deficient in antioxidant minerals *increase* oxidative stress. Those diets loaded with antioxidants decrease it.

So to keep your body's healing powers on overdrive, fortify yourself with a regular dose of antioxidants. Your body already helps protect itself by producing certain enzymes that serve as antioxidants. You can add to this protection by consuming antioxidant-rich foods.

What purpose do antioxidants serve?

The physiological process of oxidation occurs normally as part of your body's functioning, such as in respiration and metabolism. However, oxidation also produces the deleterious byproducts known as "free radical" molecules. The incidence of physical exertion, injury, and stress will increase the normal quantity of free radicals, and they will then accumulate more quickly. If their presence becomes too great, they can cause cell damage, which is part of the "oxidative stress" process. This process can bring about several negative consequences, among which is the slowing of your body's ability to heal.

Perhaps the most dramatic benefit of antioxidants in your diet is their conquest over oxidants, i.e., free radicals. Antioxidants detect and scavenge these unwanted free radicals. The free radicals are then neutralized and eliminated.

As a consequence, antioxidants reduce inflammation, which improves circulation. Tissue damage will be minimized; damaged tissue will be more quickly repaired. And healing will be thus accelerated. In a similar fashion, you will recover from workouts and strengthening exercises more easily. So you'll become stronger that much faster.

As a nice side benefit, those foods which contain lots of antioxidants also tend to be highly nutritious. Mind and body will function better in every way when your nutrition level is tip-top. You'll feel fully operational with fewer calories when you supply yourself with high-nutrient fuel. What's more, antioxidants allow your system to better utilize nutrients you've consumed. You'll get more "bang for the bite" from the food components you eat.

How can you make sure your normal diet includes enough antioxidants? To simplify matters, if you regularly eat fruits and vegetables, you will get at least a fair supply of antioxidants. So make sure you do. To really boost your system's recuperative abilities, check out the following list of antioxidant top performers (this list is not exhaustive). Include some or all of them as part of your regular eating routine.

Excellent antioxidant sources:
Blueberries, strawberries, cherries, apples, grapes, cranberries, raspberries, blackberries, vegetable oils, olives, seeds, peanuts, walnuts, almonds, avocado, whole wheat, beans, broccoli, seafood, beef, pork, chicken, brown rice, cantaloupe, peppers, spinach, squash, sweet potatoes, and citrus fruit.

In addition, black and green teas are loaded with antioxidants; so if you already enjoy either of these, continue drinking them. And good news for coffee drinkers: recent studies have found coffee, both regular and decaf, to be loaded with antioxidants. Yay!

Some other interesting antioxidant sources are red wine, dark chocolate, and honey. This does not mean you should gobble down a whole chocolate bar, eat a jar of honey, and wash it down with an entire bottle of wine. Moderation in all things. Think sips and morsels when it comes to these very sweet items.

You'll want to partake of antioxidant-rich foods as part of your shin splint recovery process, to be sure. But really, eating such foods is a good habit to get into for life. Your injury will heal quicker, but also, a high antioxidant intake will help ward off illness and just plain make you feel better. Get into the routine of consuming food which contains plenty of antioxidants, and your injury recovery program and overall health will take a big step forward.

Section 4:
Bolster Your Spirit to Accelerate Healing

Just as physical progress is crucial to your recovery, so is the can-do **attitude** that will keep you on track and feed the flames of success.

Avoid Jumping Back In Too Soon

Recovery from a bout with shin splints is quite the balancing act, isn't it? You must strategically restrain yourself from harmful activities, giving yourself a break from the source of your injury. Yet, experts generally agree that exercise and strengthening are not only OK but required for recovery. So far you've been encouraged to stretch, strengthen, move, and eat better. After all that, you must feel ready to get back into the action, maybe with even more vigor than before.

Not so fast. In addition to all its other annoying aspects, shin splints have a nasty habit of recurring. So proceed with caution. You'll need to progress a little at a time, in order to allow the leg to adapt as the exercise stress increases. Plowing ahead too hard and too soon can put you back on injured reserve status. A serious mistake is to try to "run through the pain" if you're suffering from shin splints. Forcing it more may worsen the injury and make the pain more intense and longer lasting.

This advice might sound like lecturing, but it can't hurt to receive a reminder. Persevering on a recuperation or prevention plan is where commitment comes into play. And commitment is crucial to overcome shin splints. Sometimes it entails gung ho enthusiasm for new strengthening exercises and stretches, active rehab, things you can do with vigor. But sometimes it means denial. Sometimes it means backing off. Sometimes it's boring. It's difficult to resist the temptation to jump back in too soon. But to speed healing and avoid reinjury, you have to surrender to the need for rest. If you do all other parts of the recovery plan faithfully but continue stressing your injury, you are possibly sabotaging yourself. Remember: nurture your body, not your pride.

For instance, when it comes to walking for exercise, push yourself a little, but remember to rein yourself in at the same time. Especially if you feel really revved up, as in trying to break your old records by a long shot. Walking is low impact and therefore pretty ideal as a recovery activity, but it can be overdone just like anything else. Keep all things in moderation when you're recuperating.

If you are a runner, start back up with very conservative durations and speed. Forget what you used to do in terms of time and distance. When transitioning back into the "old you," you need to do it gradually. Be enthused, but don't erase your recent progress with extreme enthusiasm that turns out to be your undoing.

Maybe rearrange your goals from what they were previously. Don't think of this as setting your sights lower. Think of it as taking care of yourself. I'd say the fact that you can get back into running at all is its own victory. Same with resuming walking, hiking, and other sports you love. Have fun, but not too much fun!

And make sure you keep up with your recovery exercises. Continue to stretch on a consistent basis. Do the strengthening exercises regularly. More flexible and stronger shin, thigh, hip, and calf region muscles will only continue to help you. Make sure to eat good food and avoid unhealthy food. Make these positive actions part of your daily routine.

Ease back into things. However humble your progress is at first, remember that you're making a comeback; enjoy the excitement and accomplishment that goes along with it. Above and beyond attitude, remember to observe the practical precautions discussed earlier.

Visualize Success and Move On

Since beginning your battle with shin splints, how do you see yourself? As an invalid? As a cripple? Or as a bundle of strength and energy, stymied by a physical setback just for the moment? Do you picture never-ending misery from your pain, or success and pain-free shins around the corner?

I believe the difference between a negative and a positive attitude, and thus the self image you maintain, can lead to very different results as you try to recuperate from shin splints. A positive attitude can serve as a major factor in a speedy recovery process. Similarly, so too can your self-image.

The body and mind are unquestionably linked. Ever had a tension headache? Most people have. If and when you've had one, do you recall anyone clamping a big vice on your head and tightening it down? Or were you hit on the head with a rubber mallet just before the headache hit? Probably not. Most likely, the headache was caused by what you perceived about the events happening around you; events that were frustrating and helped you get stressed out. What went on in your mind led to a quite tangible physical result. Your mind and body can be very closely linked. Negative thoughts can have very real physical manifestations. So for optimum healing, be careful what you think about and dwell upon.

Experiments which involve the use of placebo medications often demonstrate good examples of the power of the human mind. A recent study at Columbia University tested the effect of belief as it relates to physical reactions and sensations. Participants were administered two instances of skin cream; one batch was said to reduce pain, the other to have no effect. The cream was placed on different parts of the subjects' arms, and heat was then applied to the point of causing a burning sensation. The subjects reported those spots covered with pain-reducing cream felt less pain compared to the areas covered with the neutral cream. Brain scans measuring pain response confirmed their reports.

The applied creams were exactly the same.

What you tell yourself and what you believe may materialize into reality.

During these trying times of injury recovery, it may be difficult to see the bright side of things, day in and day out. You may not always experience high levels of cheer, but be especially careful of letting pessimism consume you. A pessimistic outlook can promote a negative self-image, and among other things increase your level of stress. This undesirable combination can progress to the point where you may feel defeated, helpless, and hopeless in the struggle against your shin condition...which in turn can spawn panic. When you panic, you experience the dramatic "fight or flight" response. This response is your body's inborn reaction to real or imagined threats, one that prepares you to fight back or run away. You would never want to live without the ability to summon the fight or flight response; it can save your life in an emergency. But having it activated regularly for a long period of time can really wear on a person. And it can slow down your recuperation process.

For instance, a by-product of extreme stress such as that caused by the fight or flight response is the hormone cortisol. Among other things, the presence of high cortisol levels can stymie your body's immune response. Dr. Frank M. Perna, a psychologist and associate professor at Boston University, explained this in the New York Times. "Athletes who are training hard are breaking down muscle," he said, "and cortisol will impede the body's ability to repair muscles, making them more likely to get injured or exacerbate a chronic injury." In a similar way, the less cortisol and other nasty by-products of stress you have saturating your tissues, the better your progress will be when healing from shin splints.

High stress also increases muscle tension, tightening those muscles up when they should be loose and flexible to help you move efficiently and protect you. Tense muscles are more susceptible to strains, tears, and cramps. And in your particular case, those key muscle groups of the lower leg and foot won't operate smoothly, and support for your vulnerable shins will be minimized. Nobody can lead a completely stress-free existence, but do what you can to avoid stressful scenarios, and relieve stress in ways that work for you. Commit to it.

On a less scientific note, a nasty bout with shin splints can bring on good old-fashioned discouragement. If you're feeling down and whipped as the condition endures, how likely are you to carry through with efforts needed to heal yourself of shin splints? Not very. Of course, being optimistic and on top of your game is not always easy. It's tough to see everyone else walking and running all over without a hint of pain, while you can't walk around the block. Allowed to run rampant, this cloudy sky engulfing your spirit could change your way of living. You might get in the habit of sulking, become sedentary and lethargic, and lead a self-defeating existence. Self-pity, which serves no valuable purpose, could take the place of ambition and activity. Many people lead their whole life without acquiring a condition like shin splints. Why you?

Well, why not you? People face all sorts of challenges, and shin splints just happen to be one you're facing currently. The condition itself is impediment enough; you can't afford any extra negativity. Don't picture yourself as an invalid or a cripple. You're strong, resilient, and capable, but sidelined with a nasty and sadly very prevalent condition. But it's a temporary condition, if you choose to beat it. Whether you spend your present moments in a state of enthusiasm or a state of gloom, the time will go by either way. Decide to be positive, remember the situation won't be around forever, and count on each day being another step toward full recovery.

An important practice recommended to athletes by sports psychologists is the act of positive visualization. The basic concept involves picturing over and over a perfect performance, a flawless execution of the actions, and a successful outcome. The athlete is never to imagine tripping up, or missing a swing, or dropping a ball. Only success. Only the perfect outcome. And with these images of an ideal performance follows the realization of it. Many athletes swear by this visualization-to-reality process. In a similar way, you can picture a successful outcome to your ordeal. See in your mind's eye fully functional, pain-free lower legs. Even try to feel them. Know with certainty that your shins can return to a stable, healthy state. And in a matter of time, they will. In the journey toward recovery from shin splints, you now know what it takes to heal. So carry through on this knowledge, and go forward with the expectation that your legs will get back to a healthy state.

Don't forget to practice the proper caution and engage in sensible activities, but move on nonetheless. Once you've committed to your recovery plan and stuck with it a while, the routine will become second nature. As will the better choices and better habits. So don't proceed with your day in fear, proceed with confidence. If you go a little too far or do a little too much, ratchet your efforts back a bit. If you make your lower legs ache now and again by doing more than you should have, like traveling down steep hills or extensive running, know that you haven't canceled out all your good efforts. Your body is adaptable, and will help you overcome any indiscretions and slight reinjuries you may experience. Just learn from it and adjust.

Make peace with yourself that your stressed shins require some significant rest, and avoidance of those factors that caused the duress in the first place. However inconvenient this is to you. Give your lower legs a break and allow them a chance to heal. You'll be back in action that much sooner.

Shin splints are an obstacle, and a big one. But people overcome all kinds of obstacles. Don't dwell on the problem to excess. Make an unwavering commitment to help yourself heal. And while you're at it, keep living your life; adjust your lifestyle as needed to recuperate.

Be confident and patient, do what needs to be done, and you *will* prevail against shin splints.

About the Author

Patrick Hafner has been involved in fitness and conditioning for over 30 years. He competed for 15 years in wrestling sports, winning numerous state, regional, and international titles, and has worked as a strength training adviser and judo instructor. As a hiking enthusiast, Patrick has explored trails all over North America and Europe. As a runner, he has completed over 100 races. Patrick holds a B.S. in Kinesiology with graduate studies from the University of Minnesota.

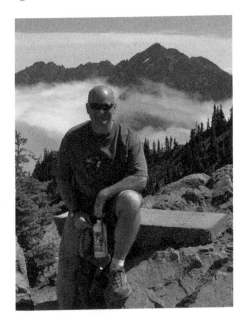

9 780980 172409